> *FOUND:* Health, Wealth, and Time in a Grocery Bag

Copyright © 2012 by Sheryl Rothert, B.S., B.Ed.
Cover Design: Jillian Rothert and Kiara Rothert
Photos: Kiara Rothert and Sheryl Rothert

No part of this publication may be reproduced, stored in a retrieved system or transmitted, (other than the meal planning list and grocery lists for personal use) in any form or any means without the prior written consent of the publisher or a license from the Canadian Copyright Licensing Agency. (Access copyright)

The methods described in the book have been tested for over 10 years as to ease of use and results.

The recipes in this book have been tested as to proper cooking times, ease of use, low cost, storage properties, and acceptance of flavour! Times may vary according to different ovens and altitudes.

All recipes are used at the risk of the consumer.

We cannot be responsible for any hazards, loss or damage that may result as a result of any recipe use.

Please consult a financial planner for further information as to the growth of one's own savings.

Printed by 1 Up Print Solutions in Calgary, Alberta, Canada.
Second printing.

ISBN-13 978153204606

1. Nutrition 2. Financial 3. Quick, easy, low-cost Recipes 4. Self-Help
5. Time-Management

> *One dollar from the sale of each book will be donated to the Food Bank*

If you would like to order more copies of this book for family members and friends, please send a cheque or money order for $24.95, (GST included) plus $4.00 shipping, total of $28.95, for each copy ordered, to the following address:

FOUND

Sheryl Rothert
9695 Hidden Valley Dr. NW
Calgary, AB T3A 5P8

Orders of more than 10, will receive *one free copy*.

Email address: sheryl.rothert@gmail.com
(e-transfer of funds is possible)

Email, within one month of purchase, to receive the *Meal Plan List* and *Grocery List* to have on your computer and smart phone!

About the Author

Sheryl Rothert has spent her life involved in education:

After graduating from the University of Alberta with a B.Sc. in Home Economics and then a B.Ed., she taught Home Economics to Junior/Senior High for 14 years. She then worked as an Education Director of a learning centre for 12 years.

Sheryl has always been mindful of shopping and cooking nutritionally, but became most conscientious of the dollars she was spending when it was time to set up monthly contributions to her RRSP.

A busy wife and mother, needing quick-to-prepare weekday meals, she found that thoughtful use of leftovers saved the day! Cook once, use twice (at least!) recipes are the foundation of Sheryl's monthly plan, with health maintained, time saved, and more dollars for the RRSP! Before shopping the store, Sheryl shops her freezer and there is the start of the PLAN!

Join us to check out the parts of the plan...

Acknowledgements

My family has been so supportive throughout the testing of these recipes and "food management" methods—I had to know if real families could live with these recipes! Many thanks to my husband, Garry, plus our daughters, Jillian and Kiara. Now that Jillian (29 yrs) is living on her own, I wanted to have a book of information for her to be sure she is eating nutritionally, and using her grocery dollars most efficiently—she has had a savings plan in place now for the last 11 years that requires consistent contributions per month, so these methods can ensure that money is always being saved!

Kiara (26 yrs) is out on her own, as well, and needs the same information. She also has the consistent per month savings plan and has mentioned to me how amazed she is that money can grow the way it can with compound interest—she is very motivated to make sure she continues this plan. As both girls develop in their careers, they will be able to contribute more per month to this plan, but it is nice to know that there is something in place now for them!

Jillian and Kiara have also been very helpful and encouraging for the presentation of the book's contents, advising and contributing on layout and photo work.

My mother, Edie, has also been very encouraging and helpful commenting on the various parts of the book for me and, of course, her enjoyment of cooking and sharing food has always been a source of inspiration for me—good times with good food shared with good friends and family is such an important part of life!

My sister, Lori, has always been there for me, to inspire and keep me going on my endeavors. Then there was the matter of formatting this book – thank goodness Lori has the knowledge to do that – here I just thought I could start writing and that would be it!

Many thanks also to the many other family members, friends and colleagues for their inspiration, opinions and encouragement! Chatting about my methods and recipes, plus the fact that I was actually writing a book, kept me going to make sure I did actually complete the book!

It is my hope that you will be able to follow the methods described in this book to be able to eat, shop, store and save to have a more nutritionally sound body and mind with more money saved for all necessary requirements and enjoyment of life!

Best wishes as you find your plan!

Dedication

To the memory of Elli Rothert (July 2008—Sheryl's husband, Garry's mom) and Ernie Renouf (September 2008—Sheryl's dad). Some of the recipes included have both in mind for type of cooking and/or favourites they enjoyed having included in regular weekly dinners or special gatherings of family and friends.

Elli thoroughly enjoyed cooking and sharing her fare. Ernie thoroughly enjoyed sharing the fare! From Red Cabbage and Rouladen on Elli's table to Roast Beef and Yorkshire Pudding on Ernie's table, there have been many a feast shared with others. It is hoped that you will all carry on the various traditions collected from your families. This collection is a mere start to continuing and starting your own traditions, whatever stage you are in your life's journey.

Sheryl Rothert

Contents

About the Author i
Acknowledgements ii
Dedication iii
Introduction 1
Nuts and Bolts of Nutrition 5
Meal Planning 25
Shop 'til You (Do not) Drop 35
Storage 49
Keeping it ALL Together 57
Think Outside the Stove 61
Miscellaneous Ways to Save 67
Time for the $$$ to GROW 71
Move It, Move It, Move It! 81
All Summed Up! 85
Recipes 91
    Slow-Cooker 95
    Beef 119
    Chicken/Turkey 135
    Pork 157
    Fish/Seafood 173
    Rice & Pasta 183
    Salads 189
    Breads 197
    Breakfast 219
    Treats 229
Recipe Index 235
    Recipe Index i

Introduction

FOUND: Health, Wealth, and Time in a Grocery Bag

If you are reading this book, you must have had a good reason to pick it up and read what is inside! Whatever that reason, you will gain some valuable tips for eating right for your health, while saving time and money as well!

I have included a small chapter on what to do with that saved money—its main purpose is to get you thinking—financial experts can then take you further. You really can save $50 to $100 to $200 each month by following the tips in this book!

This book is addressed to *ALL* ages, whether you are a parent choosing foods for your family; a young adult fresh out on your own, with or without roommates; a family with grown kids, so sometimes "empty nest" and sometimes not; recently retired with many plans for what is to come next; or a definite senior, ready to continue to live life to the fullest. The purpose of this book is to help you with your life's demands and intentions; however, they may have FOUND you!

You will find, in the chapters, as they unfold:

- **How** to make a monthly meal list, how to plan (helps to avoid the question "What is for dinner?"!)
- **How** to include the foods in that meal plan which is best for you.
- **How** to save time by choosing time-saving meals with healthy, efficient cooking methods and by adopting proper food storage methods, so as to maximize use of that food. I rarely throw anything out—food, that is! Now, with a look at my basement, you would think differently!
- **How** to get healthy by use of the meal plan, grocery shopping methods, cooking methods, and proper food storage.
- **How** to *stay* healthy with continued use of the above methods and regular exercise—yes, that, too—get moving!
- **How** to save $money$ by way of the meal plan, grocery list, and food storage.
- **Where** to put that saved $money$ to maximize its potential—just like with the proper storage of food!

All the above comes from making a *plan*...

If you are following the plan for health, saved money will be the bonus, as well as time...sounds like an oxymoron?! Really, you can buy healthy foods and save money—if you are not buying less expensive non-nutritious food and buying proper quantities (meaning you will be *eating* proper quantities) and spending less on fast food places, you will actually be saving money. Also, every last bit of food will be used, as I show you efficient, enjoyable uses of leftovers. They are so handy for replacing the need for the fast food places.

If you are following the plan for saved time, health and saved money will be the bonus…

Put the plan in place and it is easy to follow—each month gets easier and easier…

If I had put these strategies into practice 30 years ago when I first started buying groceries, I could have:

- ✓ 30 x 12 x $100, at 6.8% compounding interest…$112,000 in your savings (or wherever you think is a safe place to have your money these days!) It has been said that over time, you can actually expect an average of 6.8 % interest. Now, you might say that $112,000 is not a phenomenal amount to have saved, but is not it crazy to think that you can easily spend an extra $100 per month and, over 30 years, $36,000 is what is LOST?! If I continue to work on saving $100 per month for the next 30 years, at 6.8% interest, I can reach $923,000 In your savings, not totally gone from my wallet! For those young people who start early, they could have…

- ✓ at least, $923,000 In your savings after 60 years! I would say that is good incentive to put those plans in place for how you acquire and care for your groceries!

With the magic of compound interest, see what happens when you save the following amounts: (yes, you can skip ahead to the growing $$$ chapter to see what happens to various amounts when you put your saved money into a growth account)

- ✓ $100, $200, $300, $400; it is amazing that some people actually spend $400 more than they need to on monthly groceries! I have seen some people's budgets and they actually spend $890 a month, for four people, on groceries! Are they buying *gold-infused* ground beef or what?!

Not everyone will feel like they can give up even $50 out of their grocery budget, but the tips in this book will help you to make the most efficient use of the groceries you do buy, resulting in a healthier and happier you, with a feeling of more control over those food dollars. Gradually, you will find that even *you* will not need to spend that entire grocery budget. You *will* be able to put more towards your savings!

I have found that spending some time each month on this plan results in me knowing every day what is planned for meals, how much time is needed to prepare those meals, how much money is being spent on groceries, plus when and where I am buying those groceries. I know we are eating healthy meals in appropriate amounts, with all food being used and not thrown out. I know that I am spending $100-$200 less on groceries per month than I used to. (in spite of inflation!) $100 extra per month is always added to my RRSP, resulting in at least $112,000 extra RRSP dollars with 30 more years of savings, just from using the tips I mention in this book. If I did not follow the tips, that $112,000 just would not be there because I would have spent $100 more per month on groceries than I needed to! Thirty years of saving $100 per month results in $112,000?

Wow! That could be a nice addition to the RRSP or TFSA!

Money, health and time can easily be saved by:

- ✓ shopping in the right store
- ✓ monthly meal planning
- ✓ monthly grocery lists
- ✓ less grocery trips
- ✓ inserting meal plans in your daily planner
- ✓ planning the use of leftovers
- ✓ organizing storage in your freezer and pantry
- ✓ buying the right foods
- ✓ less eating out and more exercising

ALL of that? Do not worry—I have made it easy, easy, easy for you to follow— I know it has *got to be* easy to become a regular routine for you! I know because I need it to be easy for *me*!

As you will find, the plan to save money will also have the bonus of gaining and maintaining health, while gaining more time to do the things you enjoy!

The *recipe collection,* at the end of the book, will show you how best to apply these notions of healthy, less expensive eating, while using less time.

So.......let's get busy! Get a *highlighter* and *pen* ready!

> **"PLAN to find health, wealth and time!"**

Nuts and Bolts of Nutrition

Nuts and Bolts of Nutrition

This is a BIG chapter, as there is a lot to learn about the nutrition of the food you eat. I want to make sure you have the reasoning behind the foods you should be eating and not eating. The more you know of this information, the more motivated you will be to buy the right foods and cook the right way. This will increase your health, save you money, and does not have to take a lot of extra time—just like anything—with practice, it will get easier! The meal planning, grocery strategies and storage chapters will help to make all of this easier for you to incorporate into your daily life. Suggested foods are mentioned with the guidelines to also make this easier to participate in the daily consumption of the proper foods for the upkeep of a healthy body, for many years, without increased cost or use of time to do so!

Watching what you buy will generally result in more nutrition on your plate throughout the day; you will be less likely to snack on the wrong foods in the evening (since it is not there in the pantry!) Without a doubt, the wrong snack foods just add cost to your grocery bill, rarely add any nutrition, and can just end up as extra fat on your body! These wrong snacks can actually sometimes deplete the body of nutritional benefits it has taken in! So, you will save money and health, if you are choosing healthier snack foods over those easy to buy/quick to eat packaged foods; yes, the wrong snack foods are very convenient, so you need to make the right foods convenient as well; chopped veggies; sliced fruit, nuts; your own snack mix—have these foods front and center in your fridge and pantry. Including the right snacks actually boosts your body's metabolism and prevents overeating at meal times. Consistent "fuel" in your body makes it work so much more efficiently, which makes it a lot easier to stay with recommended serving sizes. This, then, will result in you feeling a lot more energized and rarin' to go!

If we prepare our own foods without relying on fast foods and other such prepared foods, we truly can gain health and save money—it does not have to take up that much time, especially if, when you prepare one meal for dinner, you are actually preparing two and maybe three. What?...you do not have leftovers? Who is having more than one serving? Whoever invented second helpings anyway? I know...it is a compliment to the cook and needed for farmers out in the field, but for most people: compliment the cook by saying that first serving is delicious—end of story—leave room for the healthy dessert the cook prepared! I ALWAYS make meals that will become at least a second meal—there is my fast food! It is so nice to come home to after a busy day of work! When you have leftovers for half of the next month, you only need to purchase veggies for half the month, saving more dollars! Veggies do lose their nutritional content with too much cooking, so be sure that they are not cooked too much the first time and reheated only to necessary reheating time and temperature (details discussed in *Storage* and *Leftovers* chapters)

Leftovers? Yes, leftovers, when the right foods are leftovers and reheated properly, they are great—many foods actually taste BETTER the second time around! The other day, my Mediterranean Fish Bake became Mediterranean Fish Chowder with the addition of chicken broth and sliced mushrooms—it was *scrumptious*— just like it was freshly made that day!

I like to prepare "recipe" type meals on the weekend, when there is more time. I have often found that a recipe prepared the day of eating, on a busy day, does not get the attention it deserves, so why go to all that trouble?! It is much better on a less busy day, so everyone, including the cook, really enjoys that meal, rather than gulping it down in a rush to get to hockey, ball or dance practice!

Dinners such as stews can actually make four meals—store away the other three to use later in the month or the next month for during the week when you are busier—what a relief—you have got a meal already prepared that just needs to be heated up! This way it does not seem like leftovers—it is been *planned* as a second meal—just serve with buns or bread (multi-grain) and it is a great nutritious meal on a busy day!

Other dinners that loan themselves well to being served as future meals: soups (Hamburger, Taco Soup, or Beef Burritos) can easily make four meals; stir fries and kebabs can become fajitas and roasts can become fajitas, enchiladas, soups, stews, toasted sandwiches to dip "au jus"—more ideas in future chapters—this is just to give you a taste of what can be! All of the above meals mentioned can easily incorporate all four food groups, making it so easy to make sure nutritious meals are on all the plates at your table! They are quick to make and quick to eat, AND…inexpensive! There—it is all covered! (more will be discussed in the meal planning, cooking methods and storage chapters)

The easiest way to make sure all your meals include the nutrition you need is to follow the Canada Food Guide (CFG). Guidelines for being able to incorporate this easily in your daily meals will precede a discussion of nutrition from various foods. As I said, the CFG makes it so easy, but it is nice to know which foods have which vitamins, minerals, etc., so that discussion will follow the CFG info. Sometimes, it can boggle the mind, but a good understanding is worth it to achieve and maintain a strong, disease-free body. Coincidentally, keeping good nutrition in mind actually improves memory, so this information will not be mind-boggling at all! When you put exercise into the mix, your brain will be a super power!

Navigating the Canada Food Guide:

Recently, there has been discussion from various concerned health groups that the Canada Food Guide is not so easy to follow and can be somewhat misleading as to what foods really are okay to add into our meal planning. Hence, my attempt at making it easier for you!

Whenever possible, include all four food groups in one dish or at least at every meal. The Canada Food Guide provides an outline to ensure inclusion of the proper foods in the proper amounts so as to result in your body taking in all the necessary nutrients, thus maintaining a healthy body, void of any health issues. This healthy body can then be in prime health to maintain an exercise regime that will enhance that healthy body — rather than a vicious circle, it is a healthy circle! The Canada Food Guide attempts t0 save you the time of figuring out what and how much you need of your necessary nutrients.

How to use the Canada Food Guide with recipes and meal plan:

This simple trick simplifies getting the proper nutrition with the right portions:

Divide your plate: ¼ each meat/protein, ¼ grains, ½ veggies

Since employing this trick, my portions are SO *in control*!

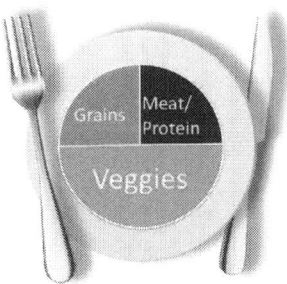

Examples:

¼ whole grain rice, ¼ chicken, ½ green beans and carrots mixed

½ spaghetti sauce and whole wheat noodles, ½ salad

¼ pork chop, ¼ mashed potatoes, ½ asparagus

See?!   ¼ meat/protein, ¼ grains, and ½ vegetables

Nuts and Bolts of Nutrition

The required amount of vegetables is easy to reach with stir-fries and salads—it is a little harder to eat a half plate of carrots!

Food Groups and Daily Recommended Servings

FRUITS & VEGETABLES
8 servings per day; ie. 4 each of vegetables and 4 each of fruits

Examples:

Breakfast	Lunch	Dinner
1 c. blueberries, 1/2 c. strawberries = 3 servings (1/2 c. = 1 serving, so 1 cup = 2 servings)	1 piece of fruit (apple, pear, peach, or banana) = 1 serving 1 cup vegetables in salad or sandwich = 1 serving	1 cup raw or cooked veggies, salad (each = 1 serving) take 2 cups = 2 servings 1 cup fruit for dessert = 1 serving
	Total: 8 Servings	

FRUITS & VEGETABLES:

They are so expensive, you say? There are many ways around that issue. One way is to buy your fruits and vegetables "in season" and freeze. Fruits can freeze as is (it is so nice to have blueberries on your cereal mid-January or blend up a purple smoothie in the depths of December!), but vegetables need a quick "blanching": boil up some water in a big pot, and dip the veggies for 1 minute, plunge into cold water, blot to dry and put into freezer bags. The ultimate way to have inexpensive asparagus ready for your stir fry—how elegant! Now, a really great way to have fruits and veggies at low cost—grow your own! For a few pennies per seed packet, you can have a great selection of fruits and vegetables just outside your back door. The cost at the grocery store would be about 3 times your seed packet cost! Yes, I know…not every climate and elevation can grow everything, but grow what you can. Carrots and pea pods are so good just fresh out of the garden! That is when they have the ultimate amount of vitamins and minerals. Freezing is closest to fresh, so grow a bunch, blanch, and freeze! Hey, it is your BBF!

I have found that to get the best flavor from frozen vegetables, use minimal water to reheat, bring to boiling and turn down to simmer for 1 minute. Add 1 teaspoon of sugar and 1 teaspoon of margarine and you are all set! By doing this method of preparation, you can use the store brand of frozen vegetables—no need to buy the expensive popular brand!

When you do cook fresh vegetables, most only need a short steaming to retain top nutrition and nice, bright colours; if your vegetables look dull in colour once cooked, say "bye"—bye to the good nutrition they once had! To preserve the nutrition and the good money you spent on those vegetables, shorten your cooking time!

GRAIN PRODUCTS
6 servings per day (8 for men 19-50 and 7 for men 51+)

Examples:

Breakfast	Lunch	Dinner
Toast (1 serving), Bagel (2 servings) Muffin (1 serving) Cereal (1 cup = 2 servings)	Bagel (2 servings) Pita bread or Bun (1 serving) Pasta (1/2 cup = 1 serving) Sandwich (2 slices = 2 servings)	Pasta, Rice, Bulgur, Quinoa (½ cup = 1 serving, 1 cup = 2 servings) 1 bun = 1 serving
Total: 6 Servings		

WHOLE GRAINS:

- ✓ aid digestion
- ✓ keep cholesterol in check
- ✓ increase metabolism
- ✓ help the brain to concentrate

Refined carbohydrates (white bread, white rice, white pasta) get in the way of good digestion, slow down metabolism, and make it harder for the brain to concentrate! If you are not keen on whole grains, introduce them gradually into your grain consumption; the health of your body will benefit in a huge way. Refined grains (white bread, rice, noodles) really do just clog up your body, slowing it down. It is just like putting the wrong fuel into your car—it just will not work that efficiently!

MILKS & ALTERNATIVES	
Children: 4—8 yrs.	2—3 servings
10—16 yr	3—4 servings
Pregnant/breastfeeding moms	3—4 servings
Women/Men 19-50 yrs	2 servings
Women/Men 51+ yrs	3 servings

Find your age above and be sure you are getting the right amount!

Examples:

Breakfast	Lunch	Dinner
Milk with cereal (1 cup = 1 serving) Yogurt (1/2 cup = 1 serving)	Yogurt (1/2 c. = 1 serving) Cheese slices (1 ½ oz. = 1 serving) Milk (1 cup = 1 serving)	Cheese on pasta, in lasagna (1 ½ oz. = 1 serving
Total: 3 Servings *If only 2 servings are needed, follow Breakfast and Lunch or Breakfast and Dinner*		

MEAT & ALTERNATIVES	
Children: 2—8 yrs	1 serving
9—13	1-2 servings
Females: 14 and up	2 servings
Males: 14 and up	3 servings

A serving of meat is the size of a deck of cards or ¼ of a regular dinner plate!

Yes, really! Meat is often overestimated as to how much we need to put on our plates. Try serving up the ¼ starch and ½ of vegetables first, and then there is only ¼ left for the meat!

Examples:

Breakfast	Lunch	Dinner
Cheese (1 ½ oz.), Yogurt (½ c.) or 1 egg or Peanut Butter (2 Tbsp.) = 1 serving	Meat (1/2 c.) in a sandwich, bun, or pita; Yogurt (1/2 c.) = 1 serving	Meat ; Chicken, Beef, Fish, Pork(1/2 c.) = 1 serving
Total: 3 Servings *For women, this will result in: 2 servings from 2 of the meals.* *For men, have 1 serving at all 3 meals, or 1 serving at one and 2 servings at the other; 2 is best in the earlier part of the day when metabolism is at the prime!*		

Suggested daily use of the Canada Food Guide: (or how to unscramble the aforementioned discussion!):

Breakfast	Lunch	Dinner
Fruits & Vegetables	**Fruits & Vegetables**	**Fruits & Vegetables**
1 c. raw fruit	1 c. salad	2 c. cooked veggies (ie. corn, broccoli, asparagus)
Grain Products	**Milk and Alternatives**	1 c. fruit for dessert
1 c. granola	1 ½ oz. cheese, grated	**Milk and Alternatives**
Milk and Alternatives	**Grain Products**	1 c. milk or 1 ½ oz. cheese
1 c. milk or ½ c. yogurt	1 pita pocket	**Grain Products**
Meat and Alternatives	**Meat and Alternatives**	1 c. wild rice
1 ½ oz. cheese or 1 egg	1 c. tuna	**Meat and Alternatives**
	Have all together in the pita pocket	1 chicken breast

Foods from the various groups can be combined for sandwiches, omelets, salads, soups, stir fries, fajitas, etc. for the total amount of servings per day. It may seem like a lot of work at first, but eventually it will become second nature. For the most part, it is a matter of making sure that you have most of the food groups represented in each of your meals and that you have the *proper serving sizes*.

REMEMBER: the ¼, ¼, ½ plate division makes it easy!

1/4 of the plate is for meat

1/4 of the plate is for starch (carbohydrates—potatoes, rice, pasta, perogies)

1/2 of the plate is for vegetables or salad

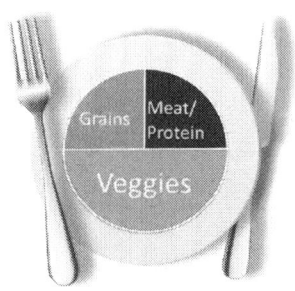

Did you notice that BREAKFAST was noted for each food group? Did you realize it is the most important meal of the day? Are you eating breakfast? What? Who has time for breakfast, you say? Sorry, you do need to make time for this most important meal—yes, really! Just think—your body has gone without food ALL night! At least 7 hours' worth! Your body now needs some good nutrition to get it in gear for the day! Your brain also needs good nutrition to get it going to support the day's activities. A brain without breakfast is not going to perform the tasks needed at school or work—your brain just cannot focus with starting the day without breakfast! Your body needs that breakfast to get your metabolism in motion—that is what keeps your body systems ticking along.

A body without breakfast is going to start to crave the wrong foods mid-morning and probably make you eat more of them than you should and that can easily pack on some extra pounds. Skipping breakfast is really not going to help you lose weight—it will gain you weight! Aaargh—where is that breakfast?! Check the list above for ideas—it does not have to take long to eat—especially if you get the fixings ready the night before. Smoothies are great for saving time and packing in a lot of nutrition. If you really cannot face eating anything first thing in the AM, pack along a nutritious breakfast to eat mid-morning. That will keep you going well until lunch. You will pass the Math test with flying colours and get that work proposal in by the deadline, stress-free!

Check the Canada Food Guide online for further information. This is a guideline for you and your family for the rest of your life! Copies of the guide are free at your nearest Service Canada office.

Basics of Nutrition or Nutrition 123 or Code VMOACFG:

The following are guidelines to the vitamins, minerals, omega 3s, and antioxidants necessary to include in your daily meals showing how to be sure all is included in the proper amounts. If you know the correct foods to eat, those to avoid, and how to do so, it is a lot easier to be motivated to actually follow through—yes, I am going to show you how to make it EASY! The recipe collection in this book helps you to follow these guidelines in an easy and inexpensive way!

Vitamin	Function	Source	How to Use
A	to decrease night blindness, skin disorders, colds, flu, infections	yellow, red, orange, dark green vegetables eg. Broccoli, spinach, oranges, strawberries, cranberries, bananas, pineapples, carrots, squash, tomatoes Also dairy foods such as milk, cheese, yogurt, cottage cheese	Breakfast: Fruit salad, cereals, omelets, fruit on the side, yogurt sundae with fruit and granola Lunch or Dinner: on the side, kebabs, salads, stir-fries, soups, stews, roasted, pizza
B	To maintain nervous system, antibody response, metabolism	Meat: beef, pork, chicken, turkey, wild fish (salmon, trout, halibut, sole, tilapia ; poultry) Eggs: boiled, scrambled, poached, omelets, sandwiches, Breakfast sandwich (all food groups) Dairy: milk, yogurt, cheese Whole grains: wheat germ, bran, whole wheat pasta, breads, and tortillas	Breakfast: Eggs or cereal Lunch: Sandwich or hearty soup Dinner: Stir-fry, kebabs, fajitas

Nuts and Bolts of Nutrition

Vitamin	Function	Source	How to Use
C	Antioxidant helps to decrease infection (protect against), Heals wounds	Citrus fruits and juice, melons, tomatoes, strawberries, leafy vegetables, potatoes (!), red peppers, broccoli	shakes, fruit salad, tossed salad, etc., potato dishes of all sorts, stir fries, soups, casseroles, stews
D	increases calcium and phosphorous absorption for development of strong bones and teeth	Sunlight—get outside for at least 15 min. per day, fortified milk, eggs, fish liver oils, meat	milk with cereal for breakfast, cheese in your sandwich for lunch, grated cheese in a casserole or salad for dinner
E	antioxidant, increases immune function, fights toxins	wheat germ, peanuts, almonds, sunflower seeds, veg. oil	add nuts and seeds to cereal, salads, casseroles burgers, meatloaf; stir fries with canola oil

Minerals	Function	Source	How to Use
Calcium	teeth and bones to be strong and healthy, regulates the growth and activity of cells, reduces inflammation	dairy products such as milk, cheese, yogurt, sour cream, cottage cheese	milk with cereal, or yogurt with granola for breakfast, cheese in salad or sandwich for lunch, sour cream with fajitas, cheese-stuffed chicken breasts, or cheese slices in burgers for dinner
Zinc	growth development, white cell production	red meats, whole grains, oysters, shellfish—crab, lobster, shrimp; dairy—milk, yogurt, cheese	whole grain toast or cereal for breakfast, crab sandwich, beef stir fry or kebabs for dinner

Vitamin	Function	Source	How to Use
Selenium	antioxidant, lowers risk of cancer and heart disease	tuna, red snapper, shrimp, crab, poultry—chicken, turkey; beef, pork, brazil nuts	seafood salad for lunch, stuffed red snapper for dinner, snack of brazil nuts
Copper	energy levels, iron absorption, lowers heart disease	mushrooms, breads, cereals, beans, peas, potatoes, lentils, sunflower seeds, nuts	cereal or toast for breakfast, salad with mushrooms, peas, seeds, and nuts for lunch or dinner
Iron	lower chances of anemia, infection, diseases, increases energy, growth, appetite (yes, you want a good appetite to eat the foods that are good for you — you need an appetite to fuel your body!)	meat, fish, poultry, whole grains, enriched breads and breakfast cereals	enriched toast or cereal for breakfast, enriched bread for sandwich with meat for filling, fajitas or stir fry for dinner
Folic Acid	lowers risk of heart disease, stroke, increases healthy red blood cells, healing of wounds	green leafy veg., asparagus, bananas	sliced bananas on cereal for breakfast, salad for lunch, or asparagus for dinner

Antioxidants

Antioxidants protect against damage from free radicals and **lessen** the effects of aging. Free radicals are produced from metabolism, pollution, and *cigarette smoke*.

Antioxidants are found in the following nutrients:

Antioxidants	Anti-O Benefit	Source
Selenium	Healthy hair and nails, increases immunity, works with Vitamin E to protect cells, reduces the risk of cancer, especially lung, prostate, and colorectal	Garlic, seeds, Brazil nuts, meats, eggs, poultry, seafood, and whole grains
Beta-carotene	Healthy skin, prevents night-blindness and infections, promotes growth and bone development	Red, yellow, orange, leafy green vegetables and fruit such as: carrots, apricots, cantaloupe, peppers, tomatoes, spinach, broccoli, sweet potatoes, and pumpkin
Vitamin E`	Protects essential fats in cell membranes and red blood cells, reduces the risk of cancer, heart disease, and other age-related diseases	Peanut butter, nuts, seeds, vegetable oils/margarine, wheat germ, avocado, whole grains, salad dressings
Vitamin C	Destroys free radicals inside and outside of the cells, helps connective tissue development, healing of wounds, iron absorption, prevents bruising, maintains healthy gums; may reduce risk of cataracts, heart disease, and cancer	peppers, tomatoes, citrus fruits, berries, broccoli, spinach, cabbage, potatoes, mango, papaya
Lycopene	helping to reduce the incidence of heart disease and various cancers by neutralizing harmful free radicals	tomatoes made into sauces and canned, as the cooking process releases **more** lycopene.

Omega 3 Fatty Acids

The benefits to Omega 3 fatty acids are many—do not be concerned about the word *fat* in there! The body does need some fat to operate properly, so let it in, but in a controlled manner—do not go ahead and have as much as you want but a daily diet void of fat is not a good thing!

Omega 3s participate in healthy cell growth, protection against breast cancer development, and the production of the prostaglandin hormone which regulates blood pressure, blood clotting, allergic responses, nerve transmissions, and kidney functions, as well as that of the gastrointestinal tract.

Omega 3s also have anti-inflammatory properties, as well as the ability to keep weight in check due to its proper use of insulin, which helps to regulate metabolism. Cardiovascular disease is also kept in check by Omega 3s, by preventing and reducing the progression of the disease. The following conditions also may be helped by Omega 3s—depression, diabetes 2, brittle hair and nails, low concentration, and fatigue.

Including the following foods in your daily meals will ensure providing your body with those hard-working Omega 3s –

Meat: fish and seafood, whole, stuffed, fillets, steaks, kebabs, (baked or barbequed), chowders, or canned (for sandwich fillings or burgers

Vegetables: use in salads, raw with dips, soups, stews, or stir fries, as well as steamed on their own: cabbage (coleslaw), cauliflower (sprinkled with grated cheese), brussel sprouts, green beans (with almonds), squash (baked), spinach, romaine lettuce (use in Caesar salad, Greek salad, or as lunch wraps)

Flaxseed: 1 ½ tablespoons daily (this can easily be added into sauces, mix mixtures, and salads.) It needs to be refrigerated, but if you keep the flaxseed in a shaker container on the fridge door, it will be handy to use. Flaxseed can also be added to your muffin mixtures, as well as breads and buns. Shaking some on your breakfast cereal is also any easy way to start your day with Omega 3s. Sandwich fillings lend themselves well to adding flaxseed—an easy way to incorporate Omega 3s into your daily diet!

Did you know that eating in the evening actually increases your weight since metabolism has quite shut down at this time of day, so the calories consumed after 7:00 at night will not be burned off, but stored as fat?! When breakfast time comes, you will not be as hungry and, therefore, will not be motivated to eat the best meal of the day! This breakfast kick starts your metabolism—you need a healthy rate of metabolism in order to efficiently use the food you are fuelling your body with. It is just like with that car—if you do not help the system to run efficiently, it will bog down and crawl, thereby hanging onto to those calories rather than burning them, thus adding to weight gain. Yes, a vicious circle, but it can be in your control: eat balanced meals with healthy snacks in between and you will keep that metabolism revved up, thereby keeping your body in top condition.

Oh, and one other thing you need in the mix—consistent exercise! More on that coming up, but know the importance of making time for exercise: your metabolism just works that much better and you will feel much better during the week with increased energy —your heart will be happy, your brain will be happy, your limbs will be happy (yes, they will, once you get into your consistent pattern of exercise!), your loved ones will be happy, your work colleagues will be happy—it goes on and on —best of all, you will be most happy and satisfied that exercise is a part of your lifestyle—and you get to wear such good-looking exercise clothes—looking good and looking cool! (or HOT, as in "smoking" HOT!—whichever you prefer!)

To help the meal planning, keep a chart handy of the necessary foods with your meal planning form—find this form in the meal planning chapter.

"How to use" the nutrients in your daily meals will be discussed more in meal planning chapter, to coordinate necessary vitamins and minerals daily—plan the month ahead and you will be assured that day after day, as the month goes on, you will be taking in the appropriate foods in the appropriate amounts. You just have to think about it once a month, not daily —you will be assured that you are eating in a healthy manner and have not spent a lot of $$ doing it; not being worried about your health or money will keep you well rested at night, especially from the exercise you will have more time for!

Cooking methods for optimal nutrition—these will be referred to in the cooking methods chapter, but basic tips to keep in mind for optimal nutrition are to keep cooking oils and butter to a minimum—1 tsp. is plenty; bake, steam and broil to increase the nutritional benefit of your meat and veggies. The use of herbs adds great flavour without depending on butter to do the flavour adding, thereby cutting down on the calories of your meal. Less costly, too, than adding ¼ to ½ cup butter with each cooking session for dinner!

Money saved: by cutting down on non-nutritious food -

$10—30—$50—$100 per month = $100—$300—$500—$1200 per year! That should be motivation enough to not put those items in your grocery cart!

Fruit and vegetables do not have to add a lot of cost—shop in season, freeze what you can when in season, and use frozen fruits and vegetables in low season—nutrition with frozen is almost as good as fresh and sometimes better! If you are not spending money on non-nutritious foods, you have more to spend on the right foods!

Be sure to get to know your vitamins and minerals: where they are found and what they are needed for. The Canada Food Guide is a good source for knowing what to eat and how much, just watch that you are eating fresh and cooked-from-scratch food. Replace refined grains with whole grains and buy a minimum of processed foods.

A balance of foods, spread out during the day, is the safest rule to follow. Your food is properly metabolized when your food intake is done over the day—not just crammed in at dinner. Skipping a meal or eating too little signals to your body to hang on to that food, not to metabolize it—it is like your body thinks it is hibernating! It hangs on to that food and stores it as fat—not in the form it needs to properly run the organs in your body!

Notions to keep in mind of when thinking of the right thing to eat:

- ✓ Health: good nutrition boosts your immune system, so less, or no days, being sick

- ✓ Organics—cost more? May be worth it and possible if you skip the foods off your grocery list that you should not eat!

- ✓ Organics reduce ingestion of pesticides and toxins; benefit outweighs the increased cost; can cut back on the cost of meat; do not need to eat as much of the meat as we tend to; buy organics at large stores to reduce cost

- ✓ Grow your own veggies, blanche and freeze for winter use:

- ✓ Start seeds inside, grow small garden inside; use coconut pots, which can go right inside the garden

- ✓ Keep a small garden inside all winter—lettuce, etc.

- ✓ Keep shakers of seeds, nuts, whole grains handy TO ADD TO MEATS, SALADS, SOUPS; for garnish and inside the foods; great for coatings for meats

- ✓ Chocolate milk—after exercise to replenish nutrients

Nuts and Bolts of Nutrition

- ✓ Skipping milk—metabolism will not work as it should
- ✓ Rich-coloured veggies/fruit contribute the most to your body nutrition-wise.

Summary:

SO much information to summarize! You have been given a mega amount of information here to give you the background knowledge you need about nutrition, but really, the Canada Food Guide, when followed properly, has looked after this for you. If you follow the guide, you will eat the best, nutritionally, for your body—you will eat the foods you need and in the PROPORTIONS you need. This will—really—result in you spending less at the grocery store. When you make your meal plan for each month, you will be keeping the Canada Food Guide, with balanced meals, in mind and if you think of filling your dinner plate with ½ veg, ¼ starch and ¼ meat, you will be well on your way! More details on the meal planning stage coming up..................

> **"PLAN to find health, wealth and time!"**

Meal Planning

> **"If you fail to plan, you plan to fail"**

Meal planning is an integral piece of the puzzle for having healthy meals available for your household, whether your household consists of 1, 2, or 10 people! With meal planning, you can control the types of meals you have for each night, whether it be a busy night requiring a quick healthy meal or a quiet evening allowing for a heavenly, tasty, nutrition-packed meal from a new recipe. Busy nights do not tend to get much of awareness from diners bent on getting to their activity on time. *No sense spending time on a special meal, if the meal is going to be consumed in less than ten minutes! The* quiet (or at least, less busy!) nights allow for more appreciation from focused dining, with the meal being of prime importance that night.

Meal planning also controls the amount of money that is spent on the grocery shopping. A grocery list is then created at home from the meal plan, then strictly followed while in the grocery store. Spending time on the list also allows for leafing through flyers for the best prices. Meals can be planned on the deals offered on round steak, turkey legs, chicken breasts, or trout. Soon, you will realize that certain stores offer the most in best prices, so you will not really find it always necessary to check out the flyers.

Meal planning lets you incorporate less expensive cuts of meat that usually need slower cooking times or marinating to tenderize the meat. Not planning results in a quick stop to pick up more expensive meat that cooks quickly.

Meal planning, obviously, allows for you to be planned for each daily meal—you can travel home from work or the regular skating or hockey practice confidently knowing that dinner is all planned and better yet, cooking away in the slow cooker, only needing some buns to be heated up! This will be a most nutritious meal, the cost of it will be low, plus there will be leftovers for next month —a meal planned already! It simply does increase health, saves time and money! Spending time each month on your meal plan is well worth the benefits of a month full of healthy meals worked into the monthly schedule of various activities, while being produced at a low cost. Being short on time does not mean needing to resort to the less healthy and higher priced fast food.

Storing and using leftovers properly means another healthy, tasty meal—it does not have to be—

> **"Oh no! Leftovers! Run!"**

See more on storage and reheating of leftovers in the Storage chapter. Your meal plan makes room for leftovers—when you plan on how they will be used and what will be served with them, a new meal makes it seem less like "Oh, no.....!"! This is HUGE for saving money, with the bonus of increased health and time being created.

Meal planning allows for buying only what is needed—it is nice to have the pantry and fridge stocked, but extra groceries in the fridge can sometimes lead to unused food being thrown out or an overstocked, unplanned-for freezer — foods easily recede to the deep, dark, unknown depths of the freezer, only to be thrown on the "annual freezer clean-out day"! With a meal plan, every single food in your fridge, freezer, and pantry has a designated use. Too much trouble? It only means no foods thrown out, which means *no dollars thrown out*! With meal planning, you end up planning your shopping trip. With meal planning, you are using your leftovers, so it all works hand in hand.

Time saved by meal planning (huh? Meal planning means spending time planning, you say!) Remember that daily trip home knowing your meal is planned? No dashing into the store—parking, shopping, paying, cooking when you get home)...yes, time saved by meal planning means—more time to exercise, (increased health benefits in a stronger body and well-working metabolism, which means more immunity to various diseases) as well as more time to get to where you need to go safely and less tired.

Part of the meal planning is proper food storage in your fridge, freezer, and pantry (less thrown out—save $20-$50; all your purchases are part of your plan, so they will get used and not forgotten)

To make sure the leftovers are used, they need to be placed in proper containers for the freezer, labeled with heating instructions and sides to serve with. (savings could be $50—$150 by using leftovers—that means you grocery bill could be that much less)

Cooking methods can also be incorporated into your meal plan. By planning certain types of meals, you can make use of small appliances for your meals—an energy saving here.

Include in your meal plan: plan for busy nights, recipes on the weekend; make enough for at least one other meal—freeze with instructions as to heating up—use during the week on busy nights—then you get a "recipe" meal, but you did not have to work so hard for it—anyone in the family can pop it in the oven!

Your own fast food—less money, no eating out, healthy food!

For the nights you do not have a "recycled" recipe meal planned, a quick meal of toasted sandwiches and veggies works. (if the veggies have been cut up the night before, handy in the fridge)

Plan meals that have a balance of the necessary nutrients in the entrée—soups, stews, casseroles, fajitas, tacos, pot pies, stir fries. Many of these meals can have the leftovers put into tortillas ready for a twist on that second meal. These types of meals have less meat in them, thereby stretching your dollars and not your stomach! They are very easily made for two meals, sometimes four with soups and stews.

A meal plan allows for a balance of needed nutrition while keeping interest up—for the cook and the eaters!

To make the meal planning easy, keep a chart handy of the necessary foods with your meal planning list—a sample is included in this chapter (include all of four of the Canada Food Guide food groups and suggested foods for each meal and snacks)

- ✓ snacks are a good thing if the right snacks are consumed; it is better for your metabolism if there are snacks between meals
- ✓ snacks to try: veggies and dip, popcorn (!), cheese and fruit
- ✓ snacks to avoid: (no nutrition—stored as fat!) chips, cheezies, pretzels, pop

If you leave every day up to chance you are more likely to consume the wrong foods, too much of them, and spend too much money—you think you are saving time, but is it worth it, and not really. If you spend time once a month planning your month's meals: no more mad rush to the grocery store on the way home from work —every day, you will know what you are having for dinner and you can just go straight home without having to stop at the grocery store, spend 5-10 min. looking for a parking spot, look for your produce and meat only to find the good stuff all gone (picked up by someone else earlier in the day), then to stand in line at the checkout to pay—the time you spent was about 10 outside, 15 searching inside (sometimes longer because you are not sure what you are looking for!), 15 in line = at least 40 min. You do not really want to do that every day, do you? With this type of shopping, you could easily spend $10 a day more than you need to, so that would be about $10 X 20

Meal Planning

working days = $200 extra dollars—WOW! Even $100 would be a nice amount to put toward something else!

You could actually save $100—$300 per month on methods described in this book. (depends on what your grocery bill was before adopting these methods and the size of your family—for a family of 4, I try to keep my bill below $500—your monthly grocery bill also depends on the accumulation of leftovers the month before! *Some months, I have not had to buy any meat for entries and my bill has just been around $250—$300! (even below $200 some months!)*

Planning meals ahead of time can ensure eating healthy, saving money, and gaining time. To make this meal planning a pleasant time for you, and not done in a rush, sit down with your activity calendar/planner, when you know you will have a couple of hours with your recipe books, anything clipped from magazines, etc. in the past month (this book has almost every recipe you will ever need, but you might discover other recipes in your lifetime that will fit your family needs and interest!) Much of the planning will be done for you by the meals you have ready in the freezer from the past month—at least half the month could be covered this way!

Following a nutrition plan, you can take the time at home, with your list, to make sure that your daily food intake will include all the best to keep your body in prime working order.

Planning a month ahead means you only have to do this meal planning once; if you can, shop once for the meats, frozen, and canned items. Each weekend, you can make a short trip to take care of dairy and produce needs, thereby spending just a short time in the store—maybe you will not have to go at all! This, then, would save time and gas! (and money, since you would be less likely to buy unnecessary items, as you will be sticking to your list and who wants to spend more time in the store than necessary—really?!) A bonus is saving time, NOT having to look for a parking spot every Saturday AM!

If you do need to divide up your monthly grocery spending money into 2 or 4 parts, it is still most beneficial to make the monthly meal plan and grocery list. This way you still only have to sit down *once* to plan for the month. For each weekend, you can have the necessary items highlighted, so you know exactly what you need to buy and will not easily stray from the list. This list also helps to budget approximate amounts that you are going to spend on the groceries—the more you do it, the better you get at guessing the prices. I love it when I pick up one of the items I need in the store and find it is less than what I estimated! Sometimes my actual bill is $10 to $20 less than my estimate—another $10 to $20 for the change jar!

The following page provides you a good list "template" to do your planning. In the next chapter, will be your grocery list that you build from your meal planning list. So that you always know day to day what is for dinner, note the meal in your daily planner—this should be placed for all to see, as in by the phone. (no more questions of "what is to eat "– whomever is asking just needs to look in the planner!)

This might seem like a lot of work, but time spent with this planning, will definitely cut down your shopping time and the money saved, plus the good health maintained, will be a giant reward!

Remember:

> **"PLAN to find health, wealth and time!"**

Monthly Meal Plan

Sun	Mon	Tues	Wed	Thurs	Fri	Sat

Use the meal planning templates to help you plan quick, easy meals on the days you are busy.

September Meal Plan

Sun	Mon	Tues	Wed	Thurs	Fri	Sat
						1 Out—sushi!
2 Rainbow Trout, Salad, Potatoes	3 Spaghetti, Bruschetta\ (freeze spaghetti)	4 Leftovers from weekend	5 Sole Roll-Ups, Salad, Rice	6 Leftovers from week	7 A Slow Beef Roll in Italy p. 97	8 Tortilla-Bake: Chicken & Spinach p. 149
9 BBQ Steak, Wild Rice, Asparagus	10 Ginger Pork Stir-Fry p. 161	11 Leftovers from weekend	12 Slow-cooked Spicy Citrus Chicken p. 104	13 Leftovers from week	14 Tacos	15 Taco Salad
16 Roast Pork, Potatoes, Carrots	17 Pork Stir Fry, rice (freeze for fajitas)	18 Leftovers from weekend	19 BBQ Honey-Mustard Chicken Thighs p. 140	20 Leftovers from week	21 Mediterranean Grilled Salmon p. 178	22 Spaghetti, Garlic toast (freeze spaghetti)
23 Parmesan Chicken	24 Parmesan Chicken Caesar Salad	25 Leftovers from weekend	26 Orange-Dijonned Pork Chops p. 114	27 Leftovers from week	28 Almond Encrusted Tilapia p. 175	29 Italian Beef and Ravioli Stew p. 132
30 Salmon Fillets, Salad, Wild Rice						

Use the meal planning templates to help you plan quick, easy meals on the days you are busy.

October Meal Plan

Sun	Mon	Tues	Wed	Thurs	Fri	Sat
	1 Salmon Salad with Romaine, cucumber	2 Leftovers from weekend	3 Pork Fajitas	4 Leftovers from week	5 Fishy Tomato Soup p. 177	6 Beef Burgers— All Cheesed Up p. 124
7 Turkey with Cheesy Broccoli Rice Bake p. 186	8 Turkey Sandwiches	9 Leftovers from weekend	10 Spaghetti— heat from Sept.	11 Leftovers from week	12 Ola! Crab Enchiladas/ Salad p. 179	13 Almond-Dijon Baked Chicken p. 139
14 Roast Chicken (freeze some)	15 Chicken/ French Dip	16 Leftovers from weekend	17 Stuffed and Wrapped Pork Chops p. 167	18 Leftovers from week	19 Tuna Burgers	20 Beefy Burritos Salad p. 121
21 Roast Pork (freeze some)	22 Steak Fajitas with Sept. steak strips / stir fry veggies	23 Leftovers from weekend	24 SO Cool Crab Cakes p. 181	25 Leftovers from week— Steak Burritos	26 Wild Rice Stuffed Trout p. 182	27 Slow-cooked Taco Soup p. 116
28 Roast Herbed Chicken and Veggies p. 111	29 Beef Stir Fry (freeze some for fajitas)	30 Leftovers from weekend	31 Italian Beef and Ravioli Stew (heat)			

Use the meal planning templates to help you plan quick, easy meals on the days you are busy.

Shop 'til You (Do not) Drop

Shop 'til you (do not!) drop

Where, when, and how you shop for groceries can make a huge difference in how much you spend and the time you spend doing it. This then will affect your health as well—if you have planned what you will buy for the meals you have planned, you are more likely to have healthy foods on your list and when you shop will affect how fresh the foods are that you spend your dollars on—I hate getting to the store at 5:30 in the late afternoon, to only have wilted lettuce to choose from, but still having to pay the price my early-rising neighbour paid for a nice fresh perky batch of lettuce!

The order in which you put your items in the cart also has an effect on the freshness of the food by the time you arrive home. Sticking to your list (much easier to do when you **have** a list!) will ensure that healthy foods arrive at your house, thus you will have saved money and it will have been well spent to provide healthy foods for you and your family!

Where to shop

The large wholesale stores have great savings, but be wary—do you have room to store the bigger purchases? Maybe you can share with a neighbour, friend or family member. Do not get carried away—it is easy to spend lots as you go down the aisles filling your cart—I find that I can use just about everything in those stores!

An in-between choice for me is the next biggest store that offers meat in family size packages that can often be divided into 2-4 meals—the store has used less packaging and time for that bigger package so it can pass on the savings to you; it is best to repackage that meat into meal-size portions when you get home, so then you are using freezer bags, but they are often more freezer proof than the store packaging; at the BIG store, you can usually get some good savings on packaging materials.

Your store choice will depend on the proximity of your house to the various stores—weigh the total savings with the added gas to get there, plus added travel time—if you do not go often, the further distance could be well worth it! Experiment for a few months to see what works the best. Give the big store a chance—it can take a few trips to get used to where everything is.

How to shop

Going to the big stores will ensure only going once a month—how often—really—do you want to do that? In the morning, the purchase lines will be shorter also—at these stores, you are more likely to have to do your own packaging, so you will be less rattled than if there are 20 shoppers behind you! Using the big shopping boxes/crates will make this faster and help with putting away at home, because it is up to you to keep items in like-categories.

Grocery shopping just once per month may not be possible for everyone, depending on the pay check frequency, but you can also make the list for a month and break that down into weekly shopping trips—if the list is there in the first place, it is really easy to stick to—I like pulling out my list each Friday afternoon to see what I need to buy—it is so nice that the list has already been made. I colour-code each week's items to make it easy to see what I need to buy that week. Colour- code? Yes, it really helps to stay focused in the store and really saves a lot of time, plus MONEY! If you do go each week, you will spend less time in the store and you will have less to package—I have found that this is a more relaxing way to grocery shop, but I do have a list that I stick to, so no extras are purchased—well, once in a while, these really scrumptious ice cream treats I have recently discovered!

To arm yourself for the grocery shopping, make your list after your meal planning. Buying in bulk—meats, bakery goods—less packaging is used, so beneficial for the environment. Use big boxes (can be bought at some grocery stores or use your own plastic containers) for your purchases in the store—no bags used, so again better for the environment and food is more organized when you get home, so less time is used for putting items away. Produce can be put into storage containers in the store and popped right into the fridge when you get home—safely stored and done quickly; meats will need to be divided and re-packaged at home—store in reusable containers—freezer-safe and, again, better for the environment! For the stores that require you to bag your own groceries, use of these boxes makes it so much faster. I just leave the boxes on the cart and pop the items in these boxes as the clerk scans them through—by the time she is done scanning, I have all the items in my boxes! I used to get frustrated with the pile of items needing to be bagged and the huge line-up of customers behind me anxiously waiting their turn.! The box system works most smoothly and I feel great about all the money I have saved with all the great healthy food I have acquired to take home to those waiting diners!

When you are going to purchase the whole month of groceries at one time, it is best to get your packaged and canned goods first and put them in the car, then you can go for the meat, deli, produce, frozen and dairy—keeps food fresher and your cart less heavy to push! Often these stores offer a discount for purchases over a certain amount, so with the once per month shopping, you will easily meet that number and gain the savings—these extra precautions of how you shop will be worth it—gain dollars, time, and with the grocery list from the meal plan, optimum health is a bonus! If I have broken down the list into weekly trips, I still follow the canned goods first option—by the time you get home, your dairy, meat and produce has spent less time out of the cool environment.

When to Shop

Plan to do your grocery shopping in the morning if you can—you will see the best meat and produce; later in the day, the best has been picked over, leaving less than the best for late risers! The shelves do get re-stocked, but it is difficult to plan your appearance in the store for the restocking time. In the morning, you will be all rested and raring to go, rather than later when you have already worked through the daily activities—you will not be as sharp of mind or your legs will not be so willing to do all that walking!

Keep a list on the fridge as you run out of items, add to the list —save for the monthly shopping, if possible.

Your meal plan will determine when to shop—less often saves money and time. Remember: the more trips you make, the more time will be spent looking for a parking spot and loading your car with the groceries. You are also more likely to add a few items, thus adding more time spent in the store and MORE MONEY!

If you do go grocery shopping once per week, be sure to stick to your list—you will keep to your schedule and your budget. (just had to say it again!)

Organize

Allow enough time to shop, stand in line, pack, unpack and put away at home—bulk foods mean repackaging and storing in the freezer, but saving money! Take those boxes to put your groceries in as you buy them—this keeps them organized through packing, and putting away at home.

Stay with your list and estimates of each item—this guides you to choose the money-saving brands and sizes. Before you leave home for the shopping trip, you will know what your total is likely to be, without a sizable surprise at the till!

Choosing store brands helps to match those estimates—they save money and are just as good as the name brands, sometimes better! With the estimates on your list, you will be confidant that your total will be a comfortable and sensible one. No sense having a crazy-large total—nobody needs or should have that!

When you plan the payment of that total, plan to pay by cash—you are more likely to stay within the budget. Yes, step beyond the comfort of that debit, or worse yet, credit card. Credit cards make it easy to buy whatever you see in the aisles and pay for a bill that can easily be a $20 to $50 to $100 more than you need. Debit cards make it easier also to spend more money. Cash has a more definite deterrent to overspending. How about that!?! Your payment method can also save you money! Cash will ensure that you stick to the list and your estimates. I have been paying for groceries by cash for many years now—it is so nice to arrive at the till knowing what your total will be—you tend to be more aware of that when you are paying by cash—with the credit card, especially, one tends not to keep that in mind so much.

Once you are at home, put the fridge items away, then deal with the repackaging of meat for the freezer; divide into two batches according to when they are going to be used in the month; in the freezer, put these batches in the appropriate container; remember: this keeps food organized, less likely to get forgotten and not used, resulting in money out the window!

Where you shop, how you shop and what you shop for can produce tremendous savings in dollars spent, time spent, and the healthiness of what you eat once you are home. All that hard work you put into that planning can be "preserved" in the organized storage.

Planning is such a big part of this quest: from your meal plan, it is easy to make the grocery list, but another part of the grocery list is placing the items in categories, which is something else that can save you time, as well as money. Make your list so that it follows the plan of the store. This helps you to buy your non-perishable items first and then the perishables, such as meats, dairy, produce and frozen items.

> **Money saved**

You can easily save $00.50—$1.00 per item if shopping at warehouse-type stores which results in $50—$100 per month. With coupons, if buying $250, for example, you could save an additional $25—$30.

Total possible savings from planned grocery shopping = $80—$130 per month! ($200/month is what is recommended that you put into long term savings, so it is possible to find a good portion, if not all, of this amount in your grocery bag!)

Coupon sites to try, for further savings:

- ✓ www.smartcanucks.ca
- ✓ www.redflagdeals.com
- ✓ www.mySavings.com
- ✓ www.save.ca
- ✓ www.frugalshopper.ca

Here is a sample list for you to follow (see next page—customize it as you wish!) The blanks are provided for you to put in your estimated cost of the items (check flyers for the first few rounds; you will get to be pretty good at this, with practice!) Having your estimate there helps to stick close to that amount—packages of meat vary in price—choose the one closest to your guess, and/or the lowest price—a slightly smaller piece of meat will be okay!

After the grocery list template are two lists with suggested estimates to get you started—prices will vary across the country, so do adjust as needed…….

> **"PLAN to find health, wealth and time!"**

Grocery List

Dairy			Meat			Produce		
Frozen			Deli					
Cleaning			Pharmacy			Miscellaneous		
			Cans/Packages					

Totals _____   Date _____

Week 1	
Week 2	
Week 3	
Week 4	
Monthly Total	$ _____

Grocery List (Sample #1)

Dairy			Meat			Produce		
Milk	2 x 4L	8.00	Ground Beef	1 lb.	4.00	Cucumber	1	2.00
Yogurt	2 x 12	10.00	Chicken Breasts	8	20.00	Tomatoes	2	3.00
Butter	1 lb.	4.00	Pork Chops	6	10.00	Mushrooms	1 pkg.	3.00
Cheese	1 lb.	5.00	Chicken pieces	3 lb.	10.00	Baby Spinach	1 bch	3.00
Ricotta Cheese	1 tub	5.00	Sirloin steak	2 lb.	10.00	Coleslaw	1 pkg.	2.00
Eggs	1 doz.	3.00	Pork Roast	3 lb.	15.00	Apples	6	3.00
Pepper Jack Cheese	1 lb.	10.00	Minute Beef Steaks	6	6.00	Romaine Lettuce	1 head	3.00
			Boneless Pork Loin	1 lb.	10.00	Red Pepper	1	3.00
Frozen			Deli			Green Pepper	2	4.00
Juice	10 cans	15.00	Sandwich meat	3 x 200 g	10.00	Carrots	1 lb.	3.00
Corn	3 lb	4.00	Tilapia	1 pkg.	8.00	Grapes	1 bag	5.00
Green Beans	3 lb	3.00	Sole	1 pkg.	6.00	Garlic	1 bulb	3.00
			Salmon Fillets	1 pkg.	10.00	Red Onion	1	1.00
Bakery						Lime	2	1.00
Whole Grain Bread	1 loaf	2.00	Kaiser Buns	4	3.00	Lemon	2	1.00
			Croissants	6	5.00	Potatoes	5 lb.	5.00
			Tortillas	3 pkg.	10.00	Bananas	4	2.00
Cleaning			Pharmacy			Miscellaneous		
Dish soap	1 L	3.00	Contact Solution	1	10.00	Napkins	1 pkg.	5.00
Dishwasher soap	1 pkg.	5.00	Toothpaste	1	3.00	Cedar plank for BBQ	1	10.00
Laundry soap	2 L	10.00	Shampoo	1 L	5.00			
Bathroom Cleaner	1 L	5.00						
Hand Soap	2 disp.	10.00						

			Cans/Packages					
Wild Rice	2 pkg.	3.00	Spaghetti Noodles	1 pkg.	3.00			
Sundried Tomatoes	1 pkg.	4.00	Tapioca (quick)	1 pkg.	3.00			
Whole Cloves	1 pkg.	3.00	Dijon Mustard	1 jar	5.00			
Salad Dressing (Peppercorn Ranch and Sundried Tomato)	1	3.00	Pasta Sauce	2 jars	6.00			
Cinnamon Sticks	2	1.00	Salsa	1 jar	3.00			
Jasmine Rice	8 lb.	8.00	Orange Marmalade	1 jar	5.00			
Sliced Almonds (bulk)	½ c.	5.00						

	Totals		Date
Week 1		290.00	August 31
Week 2		39.00	September 7
Week 3		22.00	September 14
Week 4		25.00	September 21
Monthly Total		$376.00	

*the above prices and totals are estimates

Grocery List (Sample #2)

Dairy			Meat			Produce		
Milk	2 x 4L	8.00	Ground Beef	3 lb.	12.00	Cucumber	1	2.00
Yogurt	2 x 12	10.00	Chicken Breasts	4	10.00	Green onion	1 bch	2.00
Butter	1 lb.	4.00	Pork Chops (bone-in)	6	10.00	Mushrooms	1 pkg.	3.00
Cheese, cheddar	1 lb.	5.00	Chicken thighs	6	8.00	Romaine Lettuce	1 head	2.00
Margarine	1 lb.	3.00	Sirloin steak	2 lb.	10.00	Red Pepper	1	2.00
Eggs	1 doz.	3.00	Beef Roast	3 lb.	10.00	Green Pepper	1	2.00
Monterey Jack Cheese	3 lb.	10.00	Roast Chicken	2x3 lb.	27.00	Apples	6	4.00
Sour Cream	1 tub	3.00	Assorted white fish fillets	1.5 lb.	10.00	Potatoes	5 lb.	5.00
Frozen			Deli			Celery	1 bch	2.00
Juice	10 cans	15.00	Sandwich meat	3 x 200 g	10.00	Apples	6	3.00
			Fish (whole trout)	2 lb.	10.00	Oranges	6	3.00
			Prosciutto	4 sl	3.00	Grapes	1 bch	4.00
						Bananas	4	2.00
Bakery						Onion	5	4.00
French Bread	2	4.00	Kaiser Buns	8	6.00	Lemon	1	1.00
Tortillas (flour)	2 pkg.	6.00	Croissants	6	5.00	Broccoli	1 bch	3.00
			Tortillas (corn)	1 pkg	3.00	Cauliflower	1 bch	3.00
Cleaning			Pharmacy			Miscellaneous		
Toilet Paper	18	15.00						
Paper Towels	12	10.00						

Cans/Packages								
Wild Rice	2 pkg.	3.00	BBQ Sauce	1 jar	3.00	Tuna	1 can	3.00
Chili Beans/Gravy	1 can	3.00	Panko crumbs	1 pkg	5.00	Bread Crumbs	1 pkg	5.00
Dried Cranberries	1 pkg.	5.00	Black-eyed peas	1 can	3.00	Black Beans	1 can	3.00
Jalapenos	1 jar	3.00	Green chilies	1 can	2.00	Tomato Sauch	6 oz	2.00
Tomatoes	14 oz	1.00	Soup	1 can	2.00	Consomme Soup	1 can	2.00
Italian-style tomatoes	3 cans (14 oz. ea)	6.00	Mushrooms	1 can	2.00	Chicken Broth	2 cans	4.00
Kernel Corn	2 cans (14 oz. ea)	4.00	Crabmeat	1.5 lb	20.00	Cheese Whiz	1 jar	5.00
Taco seasoning	1 pkg	2.00	Garbanzo beans	1 can (10 oz)	2.00	Taco Sauce	1 jar	3.00
Flaxseeds	1 cup	2.00	Slivered almonds	1 pkg	5.00	Whole Grain Crackers	1 box	3.00
Tortilla Chips	1 pkg.	4.00						

Totals		Date
Week 1	255.00	August 31
Week 2	53.00	September 7
Week 3	45.00	September 14
Week 4	51.00	September 21
Monthly Total	$404.00	

*the above prices and totals are estimates

Storage

> **A place for everything and everything in its place........**

Proper food storage guarantees the most use out of the food you have purchased from the store—meal planning is one step to save money, adding nutrition, with saving time, careful grocery shopping at the store is another, and storage is yet another step—cooking methods will be another, and then…..storage of the leftovers! Look at that—at least 5 steps to saving money and building nutrition with your food—it just takes investing some time for that crucial planning……it is all about how you manage the groceries you bring home from the store.

> **"PLAN to find health, wealth and time!"**

Where to store and for how long? These two factors determine keeping your food safe to eat while maintaining optimum nutrition, plus flavour. It is hard to consume that nutritious food if the flavour is not quite at optimum!

If the food is perishable—produce, meats, and dairy—most will keep in the fridge for a week. Only buy the amount of produce that can be used within a week—installments will need to be purchased each weekend for the coming week. Dairy will usually last at least two weeks—just keep a watch on the expiration dates. When a month's worth of groceries is purchased, bulk packages of meat will need to be divided into freezer bags or containers (less waste!) and labelled before frozen. Dry goods, of course, can be popped into your pantry—ideally, you have containers for the noodles, rice, and baking supplies.

Keeping your freezer organized is another *MAJOR* step to using that frozen food efficiently and not having those magnificent chicken wings lost to the recesses of the freezer. The most helpful item I began using a few years ago were three large, heavy duty plastic storage containers. The top container is used for frozen vegetables, the middle for the first half of the month's supply of meat, and the bottom container for the second half. Halfway through the month, the bottom supply comes to the middle. I also have a tray on top of the first container for frozen desserts and leftovers; the side tray also holds these types of items. Under the side tray, there could be another container, but I just tend to forget about that area of the freezer, so I keep that area free, unless there is a big turkey that needs to be stored there.

This method of organization has made a significant change to how and when I use food—nothing gets forgotten and everything gets used, especially important for leftovers! *FREE* food! Proper storage saves money—food will be used and not lost to those deep corners of the freezer—or pantry! Prepared food, stored away, saves time for meal prep—*FAST FOOD*—at home!   FREE *FAST FOOD!*

FREE HEALTHY *FAST FOOD*!   A bonus of using leftovers is **no** food thrown out—less garbage also means a benefit for the environment!

No freezer? You just need a slightly different approach. Definitely keep that fridge freezer organized. Leftovers can be used the next night, if space is limited in your fridge freezer. You can still use the leftover fajitas as baked enchiladas or stir fry or soup. Do *plan* the use of those leftovers! Within a week, you might only have to make 3 recipes, as 2 recipes could each become 2 different entrees (4) and the other recipe could be come 3! (3)   (4 + 3 = 7!) Easy math that could save you $100 or more per month!

On a weekend, it would be easy to fit in 3 recipes. The food made that weekend would be used up the following week and the next weekend, you would be ready to start again! I know many people like to operate this way—what is made on the weekend will supply the next week of dinners and you just need to rely on your fridge for storage. All of this can easily work into whatever your schedule is like—just **plan** it out and you are set! All prepared for the busy week ahead and no need to stop for fast food!

Now, for those who do have a freezer............

To assist using the leftovers and how to store - Freeze right away:

If food is properly stored (freeze right away, in good storage containers, in an organized location, labeled and planned for its use—plus the second use, third use, etc…..), food should never be thrown out again—so, ……..dollars are saved and time is saved ; food prepared at home has more nutrition than fast food and pre-packaged meals; if it is quick and easy to make your own fast food and pre-packaged meals, then you are more likely to do it. Another great benefit of leftover nights—less prep time (like ZERO!) and less dishes to wash—that benefit on its own should be enough enticement to raise the value of leftover handling in your house! You will find that good storage containers, labeled, make a huge difference in *wanting* to use those leftovers!

Safe freezing times:

For ease of using and to prevent forgetting it is there, I find it best to use fresh meats in the first month of having it there, but sometimes it is not used due to changing your mind on a meal or getting invited out, so then I try to use it in the next month—just to be sure it does get used and not forgotten. This also keeps your freezer organized.

Ground meats	3-4 months
Soups and stews	2-3 months
Fresh meats	4-6 months; steaks and beef roasts can be kept up to 12 months
Meat leftovers	2-3 months
Fresh poultry parts	9 months; whole: 12 months
Cooked poultry	4 months
Chicken nuggets, patties	1-3 months
Fish	fresh: 2-3 months cooked: 1 month

To ensure that frozen food is ready to use when you need to prepare the recipe, take it out of the freezer 2-3 days before you need it—I like to "shop" my freezer on a less busy night and take 3 or 4 items out at a time—if you are going into your freezer, you might as well take out more than one item—less trips and less time! Two days ahead is usually good, three days for larger items like roasts. The "take out" days are marked in my planner, just as the meals are. This helps to remember!

Yes, you could use your microwave for the thawing, but this does add time to your prep time and the thawing is not always even—I just feel safer and more organized if I have the food out of the freezer well enough before I need it. This way you could always change your mind about what you are using and when —sometimes impromptu activities dictate this!

Reheating leftovers:

The key to heating up leftovers is to do it at a *lower heat and for less time*. The meat has already been cooked, so you just want to heat it up—high heats will be cooking it again, decreasing the flavour and texture.

Heat food to 165 F. to be safe—

> Use thermometer to know for sure—going by looks and cutting open may have your food cooked too much, reducing the flavour—the key to reheating is not to have the leftovers taste............like leftovers!

To achieve the above, most foods —casseroles, meats, stews, can be heated at 350° F. for 45 min.—this is usually a size for 3-4 servings—for more, more time may be needed. Be sure all foods are covered, either by the casserole LID OR FOIL —TO SAVE ON FOIL, USE A BAKING SHEET TURNED UPSIDE DOWN. Also, be sure the food is thoroughly thawed and take out of the fridge ½ hour before being placed in the oven—it is so disappointing to dig into that fave dish and have it lukewarm! Fajitas and burritos may take less time—more like ½ hour.

Your stove may take less time and temperature than my mine—be sure to find what is right for you—if you find the proper "code", you will use your leftovers—if not, you will say what is the point—well, the point is—save time and money! Health is maintained, but remember—the more something is cooked, the less nutrients will remain—thus, only cook to heated through and to a safe temperature—DO NOT OVERCOOK—taste and nutrition will be less than desired. I have found that the foods that perform best as leftovers are:

> Spaghetti (tomato-based dishes), soups, stir fries, roasts, casseroles and stews. These dishes are best for ease of use and *retention of flavours.*

In order to safely use leftovers, and to the desired taste, they must be stored properly. Let cool and store in the freezer in freezer-safe containers—*label* as to contents and date used. Plan to use in the next month, to ensure the leftovers being used. This is great for saving time and money—I often have at least a half month planned using leftovers—sometimes a whole month! When you are using the leftovers, you can use as is or add to the dish, changing the original recipe —a deer stew could have the roast beef from Sunday added to it, plus the beef gravy, carrots and roast potatoes—serve with a warm crusty bread or biscuits and you have a great dinner on a busy week night! Parmesan chicken breasts transform to salads, fajitas or stir fries; stir fires to fajitas or quesadillas. Just sprinkle with cheese, salsa and bake in the oven.

This is FREE food! Be sure to find a way to use the leftovers in a way that works for you FREE food and saved money! In the months I was able to plan a whole month using leftovers every night—that was a month of almost free groceries—I just bought produce, bakery items, and dairy. If there are *still* leftovers, they can be used for lunch the next day —my lunches are always free!

Along with money saved by using leftovers– approximately $200 worth, I also saved time, since the food was pretty much prepared. It makes for a most relaxing month, that is for sure! The following month needs all new meals, so you can split the months' worth of leftovers over two months —that is just half a month worth of planning, so great also. It is nice if the free month is one of your busier months of the year or in the hot summer when the less cooking the better—a month of meat previously cooked, sliced up and used in salads with fresh produce from your garden is a great way to produce meals for your family.

If you have got your meal plan in place, the use of these leftovers goes quite smoothly—just make sure you have recorded when you need to take the leftovers out of the freezer and that you have purchased the supplementary items beforehand. More is explained in the meal planning and grocery chapters. Confusing? Too much time involved? Not really, once you get in the habit each month—and remember—FREE food and time!

The ideas in this book are meant to help you make it easy—trying the hints and the recipes will help you to be well on your way to saving time and money, plus adding healthy, nutritious meals to your diet. As a bonus of this plan, you will find that you will have more health and time to do the fun activities!

You can easily save $100—$400 per month on methods described in this chapter and the other chapters included in this book.(depends on what your grocery bill was before adopting these methods and the size of your family—for a family of 4, I try to keep my bill below $500—for some months, my bill has just been around $250—$300) Approximate amount you could save, just by what we have talked about so far:

Meal planning: $50—$200; you will be cooking your own food more, so less spent at the restaurants and fast food places; less expensive meals can be planned for, so less quick stops to buy fast cooking steak or chicken breasts; FREE leftovers will be worked into the plan; a grocery list void of less nutritious food—looks like there could even be $300 less spent on the food consumed each month! Must be a benefit of a healthier body in there as well, and there is even more ways to save those dollars!

Food storage—fridge, freezer, pantry (less thrown out—save $20—$50; all your purchases are part of your plan, so they will get used and not forgotten)

Use of leftovers—storage, labeled, sides to serve with ($50—$150)

Possible total savings from managing food purchase and use—$100—$400! This depends on accumulation of leftovers the month before—as I mentioned, for some months, I have not had to buy any meat for entries!

Imagine an extra $1200—$4800 per year! In the chapter on *How to make it grow*, you will see how that saved money can grow over the years, put into the appropriate savings vehicle. Just knowing that you have an extra $100—$400 available each month is nice, or knowing that there is $100—400 that you do not have to spend on groceries each month! Maybe your rent is going up or you have to purchase a new car or acquire maintenance for the car you do have or transit passes are going up or you have just had a baby or lost your job.....there are all kinds of reasons why it is a good idea to plan your grocery purchases. A bonus of that is keeping a healthy body—less money spent on less, or non-nutritious, food. No need to waste money on food that is not doing a thing for your body and could be damaging it!

By following the guidelines of this chapter, much money can be saved by storing fresh food properly (none will be thrown out), easily saving $20-50 per month; leftovers will be used well (saving $100-$200 per month) without receiving horrid reactions or gigantic frowns from family members when you mention leftovers—actually I never say leftovers—the dish is treated with the respect it deserves. Just say, when the question is asked, that dinner tonight is Chicken Chowder; serve it with buns and all are happy as they devour their dinner before they race off to their fastball practice, curling game or session at the gym. As I mentioned, altogether you could be saving $120-$250 per month just in the way you store your food and use leftovers—this is aside from your meal planning (save $100-$200) along with where and how you shop (another $100-$200).

In total, you could be saving anywhere from $100—$400. Times 12 months in the year that adds up to $1200—$4800, a significant amount that could be put towards your saving plan—see, it is easy to get that plan in place! Much of seeing that plan actually realized is getting the grocery list put together and sticking to it; the list is put together with your meal plan; leftovers get used with your meal plan. That grocery list will make sure you save in all the areas mentioned. Proper storage of fresh food and leftovers will see that the food purchased via your grocery list works well in utilizing time and money well, with the bonus of a healthy you!

> **"PLAN to find health, wealth and time!"**

Keeping it ALL Together

Keeping it ALL together!

In order to keep your system flowing, note your daily meals in your daily planner —whether it is a book by the phone, calendar on the wall, your "smart phone" or kitchen computer—have it handy for all family members to access; everyone has a chance to check out what is for dinner and what the activities are for the day and evening.

As the month goes along, you can be accumulating your list for next month—composed of ideas from magazines, websites, TV shows, or a new cookbook, as well as *the leftovers* resulting from the various soups, stews, casseroles, roasts and stir fries from the current month. In your plans, you can also note when food needs to be taken out of the freezer and when meals need to be prepped ahead of time.

Depending on when you are doing your grocery shopping—once per month, twice per month or weekly, that one time you sat down to assemble your list for the month produced a list that you can keep handy in your purse or car or smart phone—this helps you to stick to that list, thus saving money and ensuring healthy meals are being consumed in your household. That list can also be consulted when you are assembling the list for next month. As you shop, your receipts can be kept with that list to also consult for price knowledge of foods you regularly purchase. Coupons can also be kept with that list, as you accumulate them through the month—another source of savings!

"PLAN to find health, wealth and time!"

Think Outside the Stove

Think Outside the Stove

The use of other cooking appliances helps to save time, maintain healthy foods, and saves on energy use by not always using the stove. This is especially great for the summer time when you do not want the house heated up by using the oven! It is also a very quick way to cook meals or heat leftovers during the busy weeks of the winter! When you are doing your monthly meal planning, you can plan for the use of these alternative appliances; then you will be sure these helpful appliances do get used and you will reap the benefits for them:

The following small appliances are a great alternative to the oven:

Electric frying pan	This can also bake items.
	Be sure to keep the amount of fat used to a minimum—remember ½ tsp. is lots!
Electric grill	Great for grilled sandwiches, kebabs/ souvlaki, as well as pancakes
Slow cooker	A super time saver! Also great for the environment, using less energy, and less water is used for clean-up, since the whole meal can be cooked in one pot! This way of cooking usually results in at least two meals, so the first prep uses one pot and likely the second use as well, as it is heated in one pot or casserole dish. Small benefit, but over time, quite significant!
Microwave	Very good dinner entrees can be made in the microwave, not just heating up items. It really is good for heating up those leftovers though!
	Much time can be saved, whether for various steps of meal prep, or for the entire cooking of the meal; be sure to use microwave recipes to know the exact cooking time; for heating up leftovers, think of the microwave taking a quarter of the time as the oven; be sure to stir part way through to make sure the heat is evenly distributed
Barbeque	Most convenient to use all year round—it is usually quick and there are less dishes to clean up!

Electric Rice Cooker	This can also be used for steaming vegetables and fish—a healthy way to cook, since the food is steamed, retaining moisture of the food, and using no fat to cook, as well as using less energy than if it was cooked in a pot on the stove!
Hot rock, fondue pot, raclette	These are all great for entertaining, but also fun for the family on a Saturday night! Using these appliances adds interest to cooking various meats and veggies; adding rice and a salad makes it a healthy meal as well.
Cooking methods	Whether you are cooking with small appliances, on the stove top or in the oven, watch your additional ingredients and cooking times.
Cooking times	Food needs to be cooked to safe temperatures, to the tender-safe point, not overdone to toughness. Cooking too long means lost nutrition and lost taste.
	Remember: most vegetables only need a quick steaming to keep them nutritious, colourful, and crispy—no "mush" allowed! Using a thermometer in larger meat pieces is the best bet. Smaller pieces, especially chicken and pork, as in stir fries, need to be cooked until no longer pink.
Decorate!	Add parsley red pepper flakes, basil, nuts, seeds to the surface of your soups, stews, and casseroles—to me, this adds to the feeling of comfort as you go to serve yourself these foods—they may have been inexpensive to make, but they look just like they have been served in an elegant restaurant —it adds to making family at-home meals most pleasurable. Serve such food with special bread, or buns, and a salad—who needs to go out to eat—really?!

Additional ingredients	if you can cook vegetables along with your meat, time is saved, with less dishes to wash, so again time saved! The vegetables add flavour to your meat, as well. The use of herbs also makes for a low fat way to add flavour to your meat and veggie mixtures. When using oil, keep the amount to a minimum, while using olive oil or canola oil are the healthiest versions to use. A **teaspoon** is really all that is needed with stir fries. When you want to make sure that meat does not stick to an electric frying pan or grill pan, spray **lightly** with non-stick spray or use parchment paper. This also saves money if you are not over using your spray—it really only takes a little bit, spread with your pastry brush. This is much quicker than getting out that big jug of oil! There you go: health, time and money saved just with that little step!
Another tip	To easily add a sprinkle of nuts, seeds, bran to your foods mentioned above, as well as salads (thereby sneaking in some added health benefits), keep shakers of these items close to the cook/prep area—being handy will increase the chances of this actually happening. These items can easily be added to the breads and muffins you make.
	It is very quick to use these small appliances, unless they are stored away somewhere! Be sure to *plan* for the use of these alternative appliances when you are doing your monthly meal planning; this will ensure that these helpful appliances benefit your health, while saving you time and money!
	It is most important that you keep these appliances handy, so you will use them, otherwise sell them in a garage sale! (Then someone else will buy them and reap the benefits—good for them, but a shame for you!) If you need to, rearrange the storage in your kitchen, so that these appliances are easy to grab. It is just like the healthy food—if it is handy, it will get used. If it is easy, it will happen!

> **"PLAN to find health, wealth and time!"**

Miscellaneous Ways to Save

FOUND: more ways to save those dollars

This chapter includes a few MORE ideas for finding and saving money and health—bonus: time will be saved as well—they really do work as a team—another time-saver! If you do something to save one, you will probably be saving the other two as well!

Check out this list for miscellaneous ways to save more dollars:

1. Make your own household cleaners: baking soda and vinegar are great cleaners for many of your household cleaning duties.

2. Pharmacy—bulk, store brand, generic brands can save a considerable amount over the "popular" brands.

3. One stop shop—underwear, socks, stockings, make-up, paper towels, toilet paper, bags, wrapping ; certain grocery stores have big savings on these items

4. You have heard it before, but that daily coffee really adds up to some unnecessary spending: $5 per day on those fancy coffees leads to $100 per month, $1200 per year! Crazy, crazy, hey?!

5. Smoking—well, we hope you are not doing that anymore! $12 pack per day leads to $360 per month and $43, 600 per year! Wow—just imagine what can be done with that money ....if that $360 per month was saved at

    % compound interest for 20 years: (at least)............. $122,000!

    Hmmm....another chunk out of the mortgage payments....or education amounts....

    Incredible what can be done with that amount, or not, if it had not been saved. Okay, if you have not stopped yet, butt out now!

6. So, how about lunches—$7 per day cannot be so bad, right? Well, that is $35 per week and $140 per month. See what that website says:

    www.fiscalagents.com/toolbox/cal/invest/aoei.shtml

7. Afraid to ask about dinners? $50 to $100 per week? $50 to $100 per month—not so bad! For any of the above purchases, use the grocery shopping trick: take cash—that way you probably will not linger over dessert and coffee, or an extra glass of wine after dinner easily adding

another $20—$50 to your bill. Yes, we can have fun, but we do not have to be silly about it!

8. I hear that there are more than $1 billion dollars in unclaimed tax benefits each year. Not every family will be eligible for these benefits, but check out this website—you just might fit the "bill"!

    www.calgaryunitedway.org/main/benefits/

9. Do not forget to start that RESP, with whatever you can, each month—the Government of Canada contributes 20% of that amount!

10. Another item that might be hard to let go, but once you have, it will not be missed at all:
    How many channels do you have in your cable TV selection that you hardly ever watch? You could let it go altogether, but I did not say that yet! The cable companies are quite flexible, so just drop off a few channels and you could save $40-$50-$100/mo just with this change! That is $480-$600-$1200 a year - a nice addition to your TFSA/RRSP contributions! Less TV watching quite often leads to more physical activity, so another bonus!

Once you get thinking this way, I am sure you will think of other ways to be saving and storing away money. We have not even touched on coupons......................!

Time to move on to where to put that saved money—this is one of my favourite parts—it is exciting to see what can happen when that money is saved and put in the right place! Again, it really is all about how you..........

> **"PLAN to find health, wealth and time!"**

Time for the $$$ to GROW

Whether you want to focus on more comfortably affording necessary food to adequately feed your family and/or comfortably afford your rent and/or saving for a down payment on a condominium to end the rent circle or to save for RESPs for your children or RRSPs for yourself; maybe to save for a trip or a needed appliance for your home, or braces for someone in the family, or to pay down your mortgage sooner, then the methods described in the shopping, meal planning and storage chapters will help you to acquire those amounts—the planned use of leftovers is huge, you will find!

Yes, the *planned* use of the methods will make a difference—you can easily save $100—$200 per month to put into your child's RESP, for example. Say that you started the RESP when the child was born with $100 per month contribution—by the time your child is 18, that amount, at 3% interest, can build to **$30,000**; if you put $200 at 3% toward that RESP, the resulting amount could be **$60,000!** If you do not save that $100—$200 per month, look what could be **lost**! **$30,000 to $60,000!** It looks to me like it is worth the effort of planning and looking at alternate meal choices in order to **not** lose that money!

The resulting amount from a consistent savings plan, could go up or down, of course, depending on interest rates, but it certainly does look to be worth the effort, rather than just spending an extra $100—$200 a month on food—some of that extra food might end up being thrown out or put extra pounds on the body—both of which we certainly do not need! It is also amazing what can be saved by reducing that eating-out thing—by preparing your own meals—you really can do it so that it is not taking up too much time, so you can rely less on take-out for during the week for lunch and dinner, save a pile of money and your health, too! Fast food dinners, once a week, can add up to $80—$100 a month for a family of four! That is money that does not need to be spent at all! Once a month for a dinner out is nice, but it does not have to be a weekly thing. Lunches bought every day add up to at least $20 per week, so $80 -$100 a month PER PERSON!

So..........let's look at what you can do for that money saved from meal planning, grocery lists, proper storage and use of leftovers, plus not eating out so much:

There are other alternatives to growing that $100—$200 besides Bonds, RRSPs, RESPs, and TFSAs, such as real estate, but to me that is a more complicated procedure—if you are more adventuresome than me, go for it, but if you like the comfort of steady growth, without worry, go for the comfort of the safe returns.

A financial planner will be able to advise you on savings vehicles with higher returns, so be sure to check out the best person to work with you and your hard earned money—***remember***: a little each month adds up to a ***lot***!

It is best to get a consult early with a financial planner—what I mention here is just to get you thinking—planning is the key word here—my ideas are meant to find that needed money through the use of your groceries and to bring to the forefront what that saved money can do. The earlier you start, of course, the more that money can grow, but even when you start later, you will have more to show for your efforts than someone who does not employ these plans. As I mentioned, healthier eating will bring you more years to live—you want to able to enjoy those years as much as possible!

The following charts will give you an idea of how your money can grow with compound interest of different amounts, various interest rates and differing amount of years. You can refer to this website for further numbers:

www.fiscalagents.com/toolbox/cal/invest/aoei.shtml

Seeing what can happen to that saved money should get you in gear to use the proposed meal planning methods—it is easy to save that extra money each month and make sure it is not lost! If you do not employ the methods, the money mentioned that you can save will surely be lost to someone else's benefit, for instance the grocery store! Those big box stores are doing fine without any additional help from under-planners and overeaters!

How the money can grow: you can save $100—$400 per month on the methods described in the previous chapters . (remember—this depends on what your grocery bill was before adopting these methods and the size of your family—for a family of 4, try to keep your bill below $500—for some months, my bill really has just been around $250—$300; some months were even less!)

Do not think it is much for savings? See how it can add up with **compound interest** and see how much can be lost (lots of thousands of dollars......!), if you do not employ these money saving methods!

There have been several books written in the last two to three decades on the value of compound interest for providing a successful savings plan. It has been said on more than occasion that if you have a monthly investment of $150 (from your decreased spending at the grocery store, along with your efficient use and storage of food at home), you could have at least $2,550,650.00 in your nest egg after 50 years! (with **10%** interest —not as likely on a sustained basis, but if you can find it.....) Yes, that would be great if you are now 70 and had started this plan when you were 20, but that also means that if you start now at age 40, you will be more likely to live to 90, as a healthy bucko, with sizeable dollars at your ready. Realistically, and conservatively, speaking, this amount could be $102,000 at **1.5%** interest. Not bad, especially when you think that is what could be frittered away (LOST!) on spending $100 **extra** per month on groceries.

If you are 50 now, and started saving $100 when you were 20, with an average of **5%**, you could now have $82,000; when you are 70, that amount can grow to be $250,000. If you start now, in 20 years you will have $40,500. Mega difference! A sixth of what it could have been, but it is better than to have just lost that amount in extra grocery dollars that did not have to be spent!

I have rounded down the dollar amounts I mention to clearly see the amounts that are possible and to focus on the methods without the added confusion of a bunch of extra numbers!

If you manage, from the age of 20, to save $100 per month from these methods and invest in an RRSP, at an average return of **5%**, you will have close to $150,000 when you are 60. If, on the other hand, you do not get into the savings mode until the age of 30, you will have $82,000. You see? It is less, but better to start late, rather than not at all. As I have shown, you can easily shave **$200** off your monthly grocery bill and still come out shining like the young guy!

It has recently been stated by a major bank's financial advisor that over a lifetime of investing in RRSPs, you can expect an **average** of a **6.8%** return. With this rate in mind, this is how your savings would look (keep in mind that rates of interest change over the years, going up and down, we have about **3%**; in the 1980s, we had about **20%!**):

At 6.8% growth

Savings:	$100/mo	$200/mo	$300/mo
Over: 20 yrs	$49,000	$99,000	$148,000
Over: 30 yrs	$112,000	$225,000	$338,000
Over: 40 yrs	$234,000	$469,000	$703,000
Over: 50 yrs	$469,000	$939,000	$1,409,000
Over: 60 yrs	$923,000	$1,847,000	$2,771,880

This chart shows that if you start saving $100/mo. at 20, for 20 years, you will have **$49.000** at the age of 40. If you start saving at 50, then you will have that **$49,000** at the age of 70 —still better than not, but you can see the advantage of starting early—the saver starting at the age of 20 will have **$469, 000** at the age of 70!

Another financial planning institution has suggested that **8%** is a reasonable return to expect over a lifetime:

At 8% growth

Savings:	$100/mo	$200/mo	$300/mo
Over: 20 yrs	$56,900	$113,800	$170,700
Over: 30 yrs	$140,850	$281,700	$422,560
Over: 40 yrs	$322,100	$644,210	$966,320
Over: 50 yrs	$713,420	$1,426,840	$2,140,250
Over: 60 yrs	$1,558,230	$3,116,460	$4,674,690

Look at that! With **6.8%** growth, save $100 per month from 20 years old to 80 years old and that savings can grow to **$923,000!** If you save $200 per month, over $1 million can be reached! $300 saved per month gives you over $2 million! After 40 yrs of savings, the $100 saved per month becomes $234,000, so it is quite amazing that in 20 more years of savings that amount becomes **$923,000!**

If the **8%** growth actually happens..... WOW! It does make quite a difference to start saving that $100, or $200, or $300 per month *as soon as possible*! If you do not, then potentially, **$923,000, or $1,847,000** or **$2,771,880** is what is lost—not yours to use............If you are starting later to save, then over 30 years, you could have, at **6.8%** interest, $112,000 at $100/mo. up to $338,000 with $300/mo. That is still better to have, than not, and if you can save $300/mo from age 30 to 80, you would have **$1,409,000!**

I know that for some, saving $300/mo is not realistic—that may be their whole grocery budget and, for some, certainly more than, but for some, they could easily shave that off their grocery/eating out bill and be much healthier, and wealthier, for it.

If you do have a chance, in any of your decades, to invest your money for that higher return, then you have a sizable amount of money to work with.

Mindboggling indeed! Here is that website for you to go to check for more numbers related to your age:

www.fiscalagents.com/toolbox/cal/invest/aoei.shtml

So, *where do you* put the money you save from this efficient grocery shopping and meal management?

Save your money in a safe growth account (TFSA, RRSP) and the compound interest phenomenon will help it grow into a larger amount without any more work from you—just put in your $50—$300 a month (whatever you are able to save—again, it depends on the amount you start with, how much can be saved; just make sure it is something (!) and it will blossom!) The best way to ensure this is happening every month, without you forgetting, is to arrange with your bank to make this automatic —they call that PACC—

Pre-authorized Cash Contribution. Set this up and every month your saved money can go to an account where it will efficiently grow to become more!

Take a look here for a sampling of how your savings can grow with various rates of compound interest: (keep in mind that rates of interest change over the years)

At 1% growth

Savings:	$100/mo	$200/mo	$300/mo
Over: 20 yrs	$26,500	$53,000	$79,630
Over: 30 yrs	$41,900	$83,800	$125,790
Over: 40 yrs	$58,900	$117,800	$176,790
Over: 50 yrs	$77,700	$155,400	$233,120
Over: 60 yrs	$98,450	$196,900	$295,350

Time for the $$$ to GROW

At 1.5% growth

Savings:	$100/mo	$200/mo	$300/mo
Over: 20 yrs	$27,900	$55,800	$83,800
Over: 30 yrs	$45,300	$90,700	$136,000
Over: 40 yrs	$65,500	$131,100	$196,700
Over: 50 yrs	$89,000	$178,000	$267,000
Over: 60 yrs	$116,000	$232,400	$348,700

At 2% growth

Savings:	$100/mo	$200/mo	$300/mo
Over: 20 yrs	$29,420	$58,800	$88,200
Over: 30 yrs	$49,120	$98,200	$147,300
Over: 40 yrs	$73,140	$146,200	$219,400
Over: 50 yrs	$102,420	$204,800	$307,200
Over: 60 yrs	$138,100	$276,200	$414,300

At 3% growth

Savings:	$100/mo	$200/mo	$300/mo
Over: 20 yrs	$32,680	$65,300	$98,000
Over: 30 yrs	$57,800	$115,700	$173,600
Over: 40 yrs	$91,700	$183,400	$275,100
Over: 50 yrs	$137,000	$274,400	$411,600
Over: 60 yrs	$198,300	$396,600	$595,000

At 5% growth

Savings:	$100/mo	$200/mo	$300/mo
Over: 20 yrs	$40,580	$81,100	$121,700
Over: 30 yrs	$81,500	$163,000	$244,600
Over: 40 yrs	$148,250	$296,500	$444,700
Over: 50 yrs	$256,000	$513,800	$770,700
Over: 60 yrs	$433,000	$867,800	$1,301,800

Amazing! Just by saving dollars with your "food management plan"! Also note what is **potentially lost** if you do not adopt this plan! Crazy to let those dollars slip away!

Make sure you check that website now to plug in your personal savings amount with current interest rate and for the number of years you are interested in:

www.fiscalagents.com/toolbox/cal/invest/aoei.shtml

It is so easy to use and so motivating when you see the numbers work!

An even easier way to get a quick idea of how your money will grow with various interest rates is the

Rule of 72

Sometime, at school, you may have learned this in Math class, but it also may have been forgotten as summertime rolled around. The rule is one that Albert Einstein came up with, and once you get onto this one, you'll be seeking out interest rates all over the place to use the rule. Here is how it works:

Divide 72 by the interest rate to see how many years it will take for your money to double. For example, if the interest rate at the bank for TFSAs is 2%, your money will double every 36 years. If the rate jumps to 4%, your money will take 18 years to double. If you find an interest rate of 8 - 10% with your financial planner, your money will double every 9 – 7.2 years. This rule works with credit card balances also, but, of course, going in the opposite direction! Some credit card companies these days have an interest rate of 20% on any remaining balance: 72 divided by 20 is 3.6, so every 3.6 years that balance is doubling!

The Rule of 72 also helps you see in a very quick way that the interest rate tells you how many doubling periods are possible – 2% means that the doubling happens about 2 times in your lifetime, if you start at 20! This means, then, that 10% gives you 7.2 times of doubling. So, the higher the interest rate, the more times your money can double from compound interest. For your TFSA and RRSP, that's a very good thing! For your credit card balance, not something you want to see!

Once you see what is possible for savings over the years, you'll be so motivated to stick to your plan of meal planning, grocery lists, use of leftovers, proper storage, cooking once—using twice, food choices……….meal portions—you'll be racing around the block (lots of them!), you'll be so energized with that plan in place!

"May the forces be with you" as you do put your plan into place—bit by bit, more each month—soon, it will be second nature to you and all those in your household to consistently follow this plan.

> **"PLAN to find health, wealth and time!"**

Now.... for some recipes! …...sorry, first we will look at **exercise**, *a must to work together with eating well. Your body and mind is going to be in such great shape, and with that money growing, WOW!— the possibilities are just endless!*

Move It, Move It, Move It!

Move it, move it, move it!

Meal planning and efficient grocery shopping, plus use of leftovers has freed up your time, so now you can fit regular exercise into your week. You need exercise; your body needs exercise. Exercise helps your body's systems work more efficiently—metabolism gets revved up, and endorphins are produced, giving your mental being some great boosts. Who would not want that for themselves?

Exercise can be as simple as taking the dog for a walk, benefitting you both! Exercise makes you stronger and fitter, increasing your energy and your sleep patterns—would not you like to have a nice sound sleep every night? Exercise also relieves your stress, which also contributes to that great night's sleep.. Your brain functions better, as well—exercise increases your brain's ability to concentrate and solve problems.

Exercise does not have to be complicated—a friend of mine just found out a few months ago that she has diabetes, so with watching what she eats very carefully (even survived the buffets of her recent all-inclusive trip!) and going for a walk every day after work, she has lost 20 pounds! Walking is free and you just have to go out your door to do it!

Another combination I like is to go to the gym near my house and do ½ hour weight training, followed by ½ hour of swimming. A combination of strength training followed by aerobic exercise is great for the metabolism, as well as the heart and brain. The brain's cognitive ability—decision making and memory—actually improves with strength training! After swimming, I get the reward of the hot tub and that feeling you get when you leave the gym is super—serotonin, from the exercise, is giving me that great feeling—why would not anyone want to treat themselves to that feeling 2-3, or more times per week?! A brain and body fit for the week's activities, whatever they made be!

Do not have enough time? Well you should, if you follow the plans for saving time with meal planning and how you do your grocery shopping—there will be lots of time available for the exercise! And do not forget the money saved! Should be a BIG incentive there!

"PLAN to find health, wealth and time!"

NOW.......for the recipes...............uh.... well, first a **summary** of all that information! *THEN*, we will get to those recipes!

All Summed Up!

All Summed Up!

✓ **Nutrition**

So much information to summarize! You have been given a mega amount of information here to give you the background knowledge you need about nutrition, but really, Canada's Food Guide has looked after this for you. If you follow the guide, you will eat the best, nutritionally, for your body—you will eat the foods you need and in the PROPORTIONS you need. This will—really—result in you spending less at the grocery store.. When you make your meal plan for each month you will be keeping Canada's Food Guide in mind and if you think of filling your dinner plate with ½ veg, ¼ starch and ¼ meat, you will be well on your way!

✓ **Meal Plan**

Following a nutrition plan, you can take the time at home, with your list, to make sure that your daily food intake will include all the best to keep your body in prime working order.

Planning a month ahead means you only have to do this meal planning once; if you can, shop once for the meats, frozen, and canned items. Each weekend, you can make a short trip to take care of dairy and produce needs, thereby spending just a short time in the store—maybe you will not have to go at all! This, then, would save time and gas! (and money, since you would be less likely to buy unnecessary items, as you will be sticking to your list and who wants to spend more time in the store than necessary—really?!) A bonus is saving time NOT having to look for a parking spot every Saturday AM! If you do need to divide up your monthly grocery spending money into 2 or 4 parts, it is still most beneficial to make the monthly meal plan and grocery list. This way you still only have to sit down once to plan for the month. For each weekend, you can have the necessary items highlighted, so you know exactly what you need to buy and will not easily stray from the list. This list also helps to budget approximate amounts that you are going to spend on the groceries—the more you do it, the better you get at guessing the prices. It is great when I pick up one of the items I need in the store and find it is less than what I had estimated! Sometimes my actual bill is $10 less than my estimate—another $10 for the change jar!

Be sure to use the meal planning "template" to do your planning; once your meal plan is complete, note the dinner items in your daily planner—this should be placed for all to see, as in by the phone.

✓ **Grocery List**

You can easily save $00.50—$1.00 per item if shopping at warehouse-type stores which results in $50—$100 per month.

With store coupons, if buying $250, you could save an additional $25—$30.

Total possible savings from planned grocery shopping = $80—$130 per month! ($200/month is what is recommended that you put into long term savings, so it is possible to find a good portion, if not all, of this amount in your grocery bag!)

✓ **Organize Your Information**

Depending on when you are doing your grocery shopping—once per month, twice per month, or weekly, that one time you sat down to assemble your list for the month produced a list that you can keep handy in your purse, car, or "smart phone"–this keeps you sticking to that list, thus saving money and ensuring healthy meals are being consumed in your household. That list can also be consulted when you are assembling the list for next month. As you shop, your receipts can be kept with that list to also consult for price knowledge of foods you regularly purchase. Coupons can also be kept with that list, as you accumulate them through the month—another source of savings!

✓ **Cooking Methods**

It is very quick to use these small appliances, unless they are stored away somewhere! Be sure to **plan** for the use of these alternative appliances when you are doing your monthly meal planning; this will ensure that these helpful appliances benefit your **health**, while saving you **time** and **money**! It is most important that you keep these appliances handy, so you will use them, otherwise sell them in a garage sale! (Then someone else will buy them and reap the benefits—good for them, but a shame for you!) If you need to, rearrange the storage in your kitchen, so that these appliances are easy to grab. It is just like the healthy food—if it is handy, it will get used. If it is easy, it will happen!

✓ **Leftovers Planned**

By following the guidelines of this chapter, much money can be saved by storing fresh food properly (none will be thrown out), easily saving $20-50 per month; leftovers will be used well (saving $100-$200 per month) without receiving so-so reactions or disappointed frowns from family members when you mention leftovers— I never really say "leftovers"–the dish is treated with the respect it deserves. Just say, when the question is asked, that dinner tonight is "Taco Soup"; serve it with buns and all are happy, as they devour their dinner before they race off to their fastball practice, curling game or session at the gym. As I mentioned, altogether you could be saving $120-$250 per month just in the way you store your food and use leftovers—this is aside from your meal planning (save $100-$200) with where and how you shop (another $100-$200) In total, you could be saving anywhere from $100—$400. Times 12 months in the year that adds up to $1200—$4800, a significant amount that could be put towards your saving plan—see it is easy to get that plan in place! Much of seeing that plan actually realized is getting the grocery list put together and sticking to it; the list is put together with your meal plan; leftovers get used with your meal plan. That grocery list will make sure you save in all the areas mentioned above. Proper storage of fresh food and leftovers will see that the food purchased via your grocery list works well in utilizing time and money well, with the bonus of a healthy you!

- ✓ **Exercise**
    - o A must for metabolism to be efficient; muscles are more able to do their job, to live longer, healthier.
    - o Bones will be stronger
    - o You will have more energy for day to day activities and more exercise!
    - o Brain will work more efficiently
    - o Walking is the best—cheapest; you can go right out your front door to do it
    - o Go to the gym 3 Xs/wkWalk on the days you do not.
    - o At the gym: weight training, swimming
    - o Want more? Play various sports in the gym area at your recreation centre

- ✓ **Dollars Saved**

It could even be possible to save $300 per month, if the meal plan saves you $100, since you are PLANNING, AND you save $100 from your shopping methods and the store you choose AND you save $100 by making good use of leftovers that are PLANNED>>>money invested…more money…. live retirement comfortable and healthy: $100-$300 SAVED, then invested per month equals $1200—$3600 per year; equals $26, 500—$121,000 over 20 years; equals $98,000—$1,300,000 over 60 years; equals dollars not LOST; equals more dollars available per month for other current needs or future needs of education, vacation, and retirement! Now, get busy with the meal plan…where it all starts!

A big bonus of your plan is less stress—great for your mental health! Your dinners will be planned, appropriate groceries bought and stored, money will be saved and in a spot to grow more. You will have more time to exercise which also puts your mind in a healthy spot, as well as your body, of course! You will also be feeling *SO* good that you have this plan and there is nothing, but benefits from it!

> **"PLAN to find health, wealth and time!"**
>
> ***NOW*****...we will get to the recipes...ENJOY!**

Recipes

Imperial vs Metric—make your spoons work!
(it is pain-free......really!)

Volume	Weight
¼ tsp. = 1 ml	1 oz. = 30 g
½ tsp. = 2 ml	2 oz. = 55 g
1 tsp.= 5 ml	3 oz. = 85 g
1 tbsp. = 15 ml	4 oz. = 115 g
¼ tsp. = 1 ml	1 oz. = 30 g
½ tsp. = 2 ml	2 oz. = 55 g
1 tsp.= 5 ml	3 oz. = 85 g
1 TBSP. = 15 ml	4 oz. = 115 g
¼ c.=50 ml	5 oz.=140 g
1/3 c. =75 ml	6 oz.=170 g
½ c.= 125 ml	7 oz.=200 g
2/3 c. = 150 ml	8 oz.=250 g
¾ c.= 175 ml	16 oz. =500 g
1 c. = 250 ml	32 oz. = 1000 g

Oven Temperatures

250° F. = 120° C.	400° F. = 200° C.
275° F. = 140° C.	425° F. = 220° C.
300° F. = 150° C	450° F. = 230° C.
325° F. = 160° C.	475° F. = 240° C.
350° F. = 180° C.	500° F. = 260° C.
375 F. = 190 C.	

Recipes

Slow-Cooker

A Slow Beef Roll in Italy
Beefy Meatballs
Rouladen Slow Dance
Basil Italian Sausage Lasagna
Chicken Chowder
Crazy-Nutty Mocha Pudding Cake
Savoury Pot Roast with Mushroom Sauce
Spicy Citrus Chicken
Teriyaki Chicken with Orange Sauce
Turkey Sausage and Tortellini Soup
Turkey, Mushroom and Rice Soup
El Spicy Chicken and Rice
French Onion Soup
Hearty Sausage Casserole
Herbed Chicken
Hunter Sausage Casserole
Mushroom Beef Dip
Orange-Dijonned Pork Chops
Pork and Mushroom Marengo
Taco Soup

A *Slow* Beef Roll in Italy

Italian variation of German Rouladen!

½ c. carrot, shredded
1/3 c. zucchini, chopped
1/3 c. green pepper, chopped
¼ c. green onions, sliced

2 Tbsp. Parmesan cheese, grated

1 Tbsp. fresh parsley, snipped
1 clove garlic, minced
¼ tsp. black pepper
6 tenderized beef round steaks (minute steaks)
2 c. pasta sauce

1. In a small bowl, combine carrot, zucchini, green pepper, green onions, Parmesan cheese, parsley, garlic, and black pepper.
2. Spoon ¼ c. of the filling onto each beef piece; roll up and secure with toothpicks.
3. Place meat rolls in a 3.5 or 4 quart slow cooker. Pour pasta sauce over the rolls.
4. Cover and cook at low heat for 8-10 hrs. (or high heat for 4-5 hrs.)
5. Serve sauce with meat rolls.

Serves 6, with salad and buns

Changes: another filling idea is with sliced mushrooms and grated mozzarella cheese or with a slice of bacon and sliced pickles (similar to Rouladen)

Beefy Meatballs

It is most luxurious to come home after the day's activities to have these gems cooking away in your slow cooker!

2 beaten eggs
¾ c. fine seasoned bread crumbs
½ c. onion, finely chopped
½ c. celery, finely chopped
½ tsp. dried thyme, crushed
¼ tsp. pepper
2 Tbsp. fresh parsley, chopped
2 lbs. ground beef
10¼ oz. can mushroom soup
1 c. water
1 pkg. gravy mix
½ tsp. lemon peel, finely grated
1 bay leaf
1/8 tsp. garlic powder
1 ½ tsp. canola oil
Fresh parsley chopped, for garnish
Hot cooked mashed potatoes or noodles

1. In large bowl, combine eggs, bread crumbs, onion, celery, 2 Tbsp. parsley, pepper, and garlic powder.
2. Add ground beef and mix well. Shape mixture into 1 ½ inch balls.
3. In a skillet, brown the meatballs in hot oil, half at a time; add additional oil, if needed.
4. Drain the meatballs and add to the slow cooker.
5. In a bowl, combine soup, water, gravy mix, lemon peel, thyme and the bay leaf. Pour over the meatballs.
6. Cook at low setting for 6—8 hrs. (high heat for 3—4 hrs)
7. Discard bay leaf and serve with mashed potatoes or noodles.
8. Garnish with parsley.

Serves 8 (or 4, freezing the rest for next month!)

Rouladen S*low* Dance

The real deal!

8 slices beef rouladen	Brown Mustard
Salt, pepper, paprika	60 gr. Smoked bacon
1 tin beef broth	6 Tbsp. chopped onions
2 large dill pickles, thinly sliced	Flour for coating
1 tin sliced mushrooms	
Round-ended toothpicks	2 Tbsp. Canola margarine

1. Pound each rouladen slightly
2. Thinly spread mustard on each rouladen.
3. Sprinkle lightly with salt and pepper.
4. Add paprika to taste.
5. Lay 3 small bacon strips on each rouladen; sprinkle with chopped onion.
6. Lay the pickle slices across the bacon.
7. Roll up each slice, starting from the narrow end and poke in a round toothpick to hold in place.
8. Sprinkle each rouladen slightly with flour.
9. In a heavy skillet, heat margarine, and when hot, brown the rouladen on all sides.
10. Place the rouladen rolls in a **s*low* cooker** with the beef broth and 1 tin of water.
11. Add 1 tin of mushrooms, and cook on HIGH for 4 hrs. (or 8 hrs. on low)
12. Remove the rouladen to a platter and mix 1 ½ Tbsp. flour with 3 Tbsp. water and stir to form a paste.
13. Add ¼ c. of the hot liquid to the paste, mix well and add back to the crock pot. Add the rouladen back to the pot and cook for 1 hour more.

Serves 4 to 8 with noodles and red cabbage, or other vegetable, such as green beans, carrots, or corn.

Basil Italian Sausage Lasagna

My dream lasagna method!

1 lb. bulk sweet Italian sausage 12 no-boil lasagna noodles
2 c. ricotta cheese ¾ c. water
1 26 oz. jar chunky tomato basil and cheese pasta sauce
1 c. Italian-blend mozzarella cheese, grated

1. Lightly coat the slow cooker with cooking spray.
2. Cook sausage in a large skillet until brown. Drain off fat.
3. Stir in pasta sauce and water.
4. Place 1/2c. the meat mixture in the bottom of the slow cooker. Layer 4 of the lasagna noodles on top of the meat mixture. (break noodles to fit, if needed.)
5. Top with 1/3 each of the ricotta cheese, remaining meat mixture, and shredded cheese. Repeat the layers 2 more times, starting with the noodles and ending with meat mixture.
6. Cover the remaining cheese and store in the fridge for later.
7. Cover the slow cooker mixture and cook on low setting for 4 to 6 hours. Noodles should be soft and the centre hot.
8. Turn off slow cooker and sprinkle on the reserved cheese. Cover and let stand for 15 min. before serving.

Serves 8 to 10 with salad and garlic toast!

Chicken Chowder

I love having this cooking all day on a snowy Saturday!

1 lb. skinless, boneless chicken breasts, cubed
11 oz. kernel corn, frozen
1 4 oz. tin diced green chilies
¼ c. taco seasoning
1 c. sour cream
1 red pepper, diced
1 tin condensed potato soup
2 Tbsp. fresh cilantro
3 c. chicken broth
4 oz. Jalapeno Cheese Spread

1. In a **crock pot (s*low* cooker)**, combine: chicken, corn, soup, undrained chili peppers, cilantro, and taco seasoning; mix.
2. Stir in chicken broth and cook on low for 6 hrs. (or high for 3 hrs.)
3. One half hour before the chowder is ready, stir in the jalapeno spread and sour cream; stir to combine
4. When ready, "decorate" with parsley flakes and crushed red pepper flakes

Serves 6, with French Onion biscuits.

---

*Freeze chowder leftovers; this is **great** heated up! This soup makes it easy to use any leftover corn, rice, chicken kebabs, chicken stir fry, or chicken fajitas!*

Crazy-Nutty Mocha Pudding Cake

Yum—dessert in the slow cooker—cozy reward for enduring a COL-D-D-D day!

1 c. all-purpose flour
½ c. sugar
2 Tbsp. cocoa powder
1 ½ tsp. baking powder
½ c. milk
2 Tbsp. butter, melted
½ c. miniature semisweet chocolate pieces
¼ c. coffee liqueur (optional)

½ c. pecans, chopped
¾ c. sugar
¼ c. cocoa powder
1 Tbsp. instant coffee crystals
1 ½ c. boiling water
1 tsp. vanilla

1. In a bowl, combine: flour, ½ c. sugar, 2 Tbsp. cocoa, and baking powder. Add milk, melted butter, and vanilla.
2. Stir until batter is smooth; add chocolate pieces and pecans.
3. Spread batter evenly on the bottom of a 3 ½—4 quart slow cooker.
4. In a small bowl, combine the ¾ c. sugar and ¼ c. cocoa; in a liquid measuring cup, dissolve coffee crystals in the boiling water and stir in the liqueur, if using.
5. Gradually stir the sugar-cocoa mixture into the coffee mixture.
6. Pour the mixture evenly over the batter in the slow cooker.
7. Cover; cook on high setting for 2½ hrs. (center will appear moist, but will set on standing)
8. Let stand 30 min. to cool slightly before serving.
9. To serve, spoon warm cake into dessert dishes, spoon pudding over cake, and follow with a scoop of vanilla ice cream.

Serves 8

Savoury Pot Roast with Mushroom Sauce

Great way to get your Sunday dinner prepared early in the day!

1.5 lb (3 kg) boneless eye of round or rump roast
4 med. potatoes, quartered   1 can golden mushroom soup
2 c. carrots, cut into 1 ½" pieces   ½ tsp. basil, crushed

1. Trim fat from roast.
2. Lightly coat a large skillet with canola spray. Heat over med. heat and brown all sides of the roast.
3. Place potatoes and carrots in the slow cooker. Place browned roast over the vegetables.
4. In a small bowl, combine the basil with the soup; pour over the roast.
5. Cover and cook on low setting for 10-12 hrs. (high for 5-6 hrs.)
6. To serve, place sliced meat with vegetables on a platter and pass the sauce!

Serves 5—6: for a complete dinner or you could also add a salad.

Spicy Citrus Chicken

Comforting tang!

6 oz. can frozen pineapple-orange juice concentrate, thawed

½ c. ketchup

2 Tbsp. lemon juice

¼ tsp. cayenne

1 Tbsp. quick-cooking tapioca

2 ½ to 3 pounds chicken pieces, skinned

Hot cooked rice

2 sticks cinnamon

8 whole allspice

4 whole cloves

1. For sauce, combine in a small bowl: juice concentrate, ketchup, lemon juice, and cayenne. Pour half the sauce into the slow cooker.
2. Add tapioca and stir.
3. For spice bag: place cinnamon, allspice and cloves in a 100% cotton cheesecloth and tie closed with a clean kitchen string. Add bag to the cooker with chicken pieces.
4. Pour remaining sauce over the chicken.
5. Cover and cook on low-heat setting for 8-9 hours (or on high for 4-4 ½ hours)
6. Transfer chicken to serving platter, reserving sauce.
7. Discard spice bag. Strain sauce and skim off the fat. Serve sauce and hot rice with the chicken.

Serves 4 with salad or veggies with buns.

Teriyaki Chicken with Orange Sauce

With protein and veggies, all you need is rice!

1 pound skinless, boneless chicken breast halves, or thighs
1 16 oz. pkg. frozen mix of broccoli, carrots, and water chestnuts

2 Tbsp. quick-cooking tapioca	1 tsp. dry mustard
¼ c. chicken broth	1/2 tsp. ground ginger
3 Tbsp. orange marmalade	2 Tbsp. teriyaki sauce

2 cups hot cooked rice

8. Cut chicken into 1 inch pieces; set aside.
9. Place frozen vegetables in slow cooker and sprinkle tapioca over; stir to combine.
10. Place chicken over vegetables.
11. For sauce, combine in a small bowl: chicken broth, marmalade, teriyaki sauce, mustard, and ginger. Pour sauce over chicken pieces.
12. Cover and cook on low heat setting for 4-5 hours (or high for 2-2 ½ hours)

Serves 4 with rice!

Turkey Sausage and Tortellini Soup

Another very good and VERY EASY soup!

6 oz. cooked, smoked turkey (or ham) sausage, sliced)
2 c. coleslaw mix
1 green pepper, chopped
2 14 oz. cans stewed tomatoes
Grated Parmesan cheese
1 can French onion soup
3 c. water
9 oz. package cheese-filled tortellini
2 tsp. each basil and oregano

1. Place in the Slow-Cooker: sausage, coleslaw mix, undrained tomatoes, soup, and water.
2. Cover and cook on low heat for 8—10 hours (or on high heat for 4—5 hours)
3. At end of cooking time, if using low heat, turn to high heat and stir in tortellini with green peppers. Cover and cook for 15 min. more.
4. Ladle soup into bowls and sprinkle with Parmesan cheese.

Serves 6 with a great foccacia!

Turkey, Mushroom and Rice Soup

A wonderful Asian flavour!

2 c. fresh mushrooms, sliced	2 Tbsp. soy sauce
1 ½ c. bok choy, sliced	1 Tbsp. sesame oil
1 med. onion, chopped	4 cloves garlic, minced
2 med. carrots, sliced	2 tsp. fresh ginger, grated
1 lb. turkey breast, cut into 1" pieces	1 c. instant rice
3 c. chicken broth	

1. In the Slow-Cooker, place: mushrooms, bok choy, onion, and carrots. Add the turkey.
2. Combine in small bowl: chicken broth, soy sauce, sesame oil, garlic, and ginger. Pour over the vegetables and turkey.
3. Cover and cook on low-heat for 8 to 10 hours (or on high for 4 to 5 hours)
4. At the end of cooking time, stir in the rice, cover and let stand for 10 min. Ladle into bowls.

Serves 6 with bean sprouts, peppers, and mint leaves to garnish.

Changes: use chicken or pork in place of the turkey.

El Spicy Chicken and Rice

So easy—prep the night before, turn on in the AM, and you have got a super dinner to come home to!

1 lb. boneless, skinless chicken thighs, cut into ¾" pieces
1 ½ c. uncooked long-grain rice   ¼ c. chopped green chilies
1 c. chunky salsa   1 c. sour cream
1 ¾ c. chicken broth
1 c. shredded Monterey Jack cheese

1. In Slow-Cooker, mix chicken, rice, salsa, broth and chilies.
2. Cover and cook on **low** setting for 6 to 7 hours.
3. At 5 minutes before serving, turn off heat; stir in sour cream and **half** of the cheese. Sprinkle remaining cheese over top.
4. Cover and let stand 5 minutes.
5. Serve with additional salsa on the side.

Serves 4 with salad or green vegetable and buns.

Leftovers could be rolled up in tortillas for the second meal:

Place in glass baking dish, sprayed with canola spray, top with salsa and grated cheese; freeze for later. Heat at 350°F., covered with foil, for ½ hour. Great for lunches also!

French Onion Soup

A definite cozy addition to a winter day's meal!

4—6 onions, thinly sliced	1 ½ tsp. Worcestershire sauce
1 clove garlic, minced	1/8 tsp. pepper
3 Tbsp. margarine	6—8 of 1 inch slices French bread
4 ½ c. beef broth	
6—8 ¾ oz. slices Swiss or Gruyere cheese	

1. In a large skillet, fry onions and garlic in hot margarine, covered, over medium-low heat for 20 min. or until tender, stirring occasionally.
2. Transfer onion mixture to a slow cooker. Add beef broth, Worcestershire sauce, and pepper.
3. Cover and cook for 2 ½ to 3 hours, on HIGH.
4. Before serving soup, toast bread slices. Arrange bread slices on a baking sheet, top each with a cheese slice and broil for 2—3 min., or until cheese is light brown and bubbly.
5. Ladle soup into bowls and top with cheese toast.

Serves 6—8 with spinach salad or as appetizer to Sunday dinner.

Second use: add to Hamburger Soup or take to lunch with some of the salad.

Hearty Sausage Casserole

So good on a cool Fall day!

2 pkg. beef gravy mix	1 (14 oz.) can stewed tomatoes
2 Tbsp. Italian dressing	1 Tbsp. Dijon mustard
1 lb. smoked sausage, cut into 1" pieces	¼ c. each of chopped green
2 c. quartered red potatoes	pepper, celery, and onion
2 Tbsp. cornstarch	5 c. hot water

1. Place all ingredients, except the cornstarch, into a slow cooker.
2. Cover; cook on low setting for 8 to 10 hours (or on high for 4-5 hrs)
3. One half hour before serving, remove one ladle of hot liquid and mix with the cornstarch. Place back into the sausage mixture and turn the heat to high. This will thicken the gravy

Serves 8 with crusty buns or the "Italian-French Bread".

---
*This dish freezes well to be used next month!
For soup, add 1 to 2 cups beef broth.*

Herbed Chicken

Very good and VERY EASY!

8 oz. fresh mushrooms, halved	½ tsp. dried thyme, crushed
16 pearl onions, peeled	¼ tsp. black pepper
½ c. chicken broth	1 bay leaf
¼ c. dry red wine	4 chicken parts, skinned
2 Tbsp. tomato paste	¼ c. chicken broth
½ tsp. garlic powder	2 Tbsp. flour
½ tsp. dried rosemary, crushed	Fresh parsley, chopped

1. Place mushrooms and onions in the slow cooker.
2. Stir in the broth, wine, tomato paste, garlic powder, rosemary, thyme, pepper, and bay leaf. Add the chicken pieces.
3. Cook at low setting for 7—8 hrs. (or on high for 3.5-4 hrs)
4. Transfer chicken and vegetables to serving platter with a slotted spoon and discard bay leaf. Cover chicken and vegetables to keep warm.
5. To make a sauce: skim fat from cooking liquid. Measure 2 c. of the liquid, adding additional chicken broth, if needed, to equal 2 c.
6. Transfer liquid to a medium saucepan. In a small bowl, stir the ¼ c. broth into the flour and stir into mixture in the saucepan.
7. Cook and stir until thickened and bubbly; cook and stir for 1 min. more. Spoon some of the sauce over the chicken and pass the rest in serving dish.

Serves 4 with mashed potatoes or rice, and green beans.

Hunter Sausage Casserole

Prepare one winter's night before a busy day, turn on in the morning, and supper is all set for when you arrive home after the day's activities!

2 pkg. gravy mix	1 can stewed tomatoes
1 ring of cooked, smoked sausage	3 Tbsp. Italian dressing
5 c. hot water	1 Tbsp. Dijon mustard
2 c. chopped cabbage	2 c. quartered red potatoes

¼ c. cornstarch (mix with some of the hot water before adding)

1. Add all ingredients to the Slow-Cooker; stir until mixed well.
2. Cover, cook on *low* heat for 8 to 10 hrs (or high for 4-5 hrs)
3. Half hour before serving—if sauce is not thick enough, take out ½ c. of broth and mix with 2 Tbsp. cornstarch; add back to the slow cooker.

Serves 8 with buns.

Chopped green pepper could be used instead of the cabbage, or in addition to—just add in the last ½ hr. to keep that nice green colour!

Freezes well for the second time around!

Mushroom Beef Dip

So nice to come home to after a busy activity-packed day!

1 3 lb. beef round or rump roast
4 portobello mushrooms, split
1 ¾ c. beef broth
8 Kaiser buns, split, toasted
1 large red onion, sliced

1. Trim fat from roast and brown meat on all sides in hot oil in large skillet. Drain fat and place roast in slow cooker.
2. Clean mushrooms, discard stems. Cut mushrooms into ¼" slices and add to cooker.
3. Pour broth over meat and mushrooms.
4. Cook on low heat for 8-9 hours (or on high for 4-4 ½ hours)
5. Remove meat from cooker and let stand for 10 min.
6. Remove mushrooms with slotted spoon and set aside. Thinly slice meat, then arrange meat, mushrooms, and onions on buns.
7. Pour cooking juices into measuring cup and skim off juices. Pour the juice into individual bowls for dipping.
8. Serve the buns with tops and the bowls for dipping.

Serves 8 with veggies and dip or a salad, such as coleslaw

Orange-Dijonned Pork Chops

A slow-cooked delicacy!

6 boneless pork loin chops
Salt and pepper
½ tsp. thyme

1 c. orange marmalade
1/3 c. Dijon mustard

1. Sprinkle both sides of the chops, lightly, with salt and pepper; place chops in the Slow-Cooker.
2. Combine orange marmalade and mustard in a small bowl.
3. Remove 2 Tbsp. of the marmalade mixture and keep in the fridge.
4. Combine remaining mixture with ¼ c. water and pour over chops.
5. Cover and cook on low for 6—7 hours (or on high for 3—3.5 hours)

Serve pork chops with reserved sauce.

Serves 6 with wild rice and salad, or asparagus.

Pork and Mushroom Marengo

A great "dance" on a cool, busy day!

1 ½ lb. boneless pork shoulder, cut into 1" cubes

1 Tbsp. canola oil	½ tsp. dried thyme, crushed
8 oz. fresh mushrooms, sliced	1 tsp. instant chicken bouillon
1 med. onion, chopped	¼ tsp. salt
1 14 oz. can diced tomatoes	Dash of pepper
1 c. water	1/3 c. cold water
1 Tbsp. dried marjoram crushed	3 Tbsp. flour
2 c. hot cooked rice	

1. In a large skillet, brown the meat, half at a time, in hot oil. Drain the fat.
2. In slow cooker, place the mushrooms, onion, and meat.
3. In a bowl, combine *undrained* tomatoes, 1 c. water, marjoram, thyme, bouillon, salt, and pepper. Pour over mixture in slow cooker.
4. Cover, and cook on low setting for 8-10 hours (or high heat for 4-5 hours.)
5. If using low-heat setting, turn to high. In a bowl, combine the ½ c. flour and 1/3 c. cold water. Stir flour mixture into pork mixture in the slow cooker. Cover and cook on high setting for 15—20 min., or until thickened.
6. Serve over hot rice.

Serves 4 with salad or green vegetable such as asparagus, or add green beans to the recipe

Second use: Add more beef broth for soup or serve over buns as is.

Taco Soup

Many beans for many nutritious bites—do not worry—they taste excellent with the zesty ingredients!

1 lb. ground beef	1 15 oz. can garbonzo beans
1 15 oz. can black-eyed peas,	1 14.5 oz. spicy tomatoes, undrained
1 15 oz. can black beans, undrained	1 small can green chilies
1 11 oz. can kernel corn	
1 15 oz. chili beans with gravy	1 pkg. taco seasoning
Sour cream	Tortilla chips

1. In large skillet, cook ground beef until brown.
2. In slow cooker, combine ground beef, black-eyed peas, black beans, chili beans, garbonzo beans, tomatoes, chilies, and corn.
3. Add the taco seasoning; stir well to combine.
4. Cover; cook on low heat for 6-8 hrs. (on high for 3-4 hrs.)

Serves 8 with sour cream and tortilla chips; add some great jalapeno cheese bread!

Freezes and heats up well—both first and second use are so nice to come home to during a busy week! Also works great on a wintery Saturday!

Beef

Beef Burgers—All Cheesed-Up!

Beef Fajitas BBQ Flavour

Tanged up Beef Patties

Beefy Burritos

Cheddar Beef Tortiere

Cheesy Beef Burgers

Coffee-Seasoned Steaks

Easier than Lasagna Burgers

Great Caesar Burgers

Truly Divine Meatloaf

Italian Beef and Ravioli Stew

Zesty Taco Pie

Beef Burgers—All Cheesed-Up!

Packed with flavour, these burgers!

1 lb. extra-lean ground beef
¼ c. cheese of choice, grated
½ c. fresh bread crumbs
¼ c. BBQ sauce, divided
4 burger buns

1. Preheat BBQ to med-high heat.
2. Mix meat with cheese, bread crumbs, and 2 Tbsp. of BBQ sauce.
3. Shape mixture into 4 patties.
4. Place patties on the BBQ; cover with BBQ lid. Grill 4-6 min. on each side or until burgers are cooked through (160 F.), brushing with remaining 2 Tbsp. of BBQ sauce during the last 2 min. of grilling time.
5. Fill buns with burgers and fixings such as lettuce, tomato, onion.

Serves 4 with raw veggies

Beef Fajitas BBQ Flavour

So easy............so good!

1 Tbsp. canola oil	1 onion, sliced
1 lb. sirloin steak, cut into strips	½ c. BBQ sauce
1 red pepper, cut into strips	8 flour tortillas
1 green pepper, cut into strips	1 c. sliced mushrooms

1. Heat oil in large skillet over med-high heat.
2. Add beef, mushrooms and onions—cook and stir 10 min.—until meat is cooked through and onions are opaque.
3. Add peppers with BBQ sauce and mix well—turn heat down to med-low; cook 5 min. more to have peppers still crisp.
4. Serve in tortillas or over rice.

Serves 4 with 1 tortilla each and 4 to freeze.

Fresh veggies on the side are always good!

This recipe can be also be used as a stir fry served over rice, rather than wrapped in tortillas; if there are leftovers, wrap them in tortillas to be ready for the 2nd use! Great for lunches, too!

Tanged up Beef Patties

Freeze easily when made ahead and so easy to cook once you are ready!

1 large egg	1 c. onion, finely chopped
1/3 c. milk	1 tsp. salt
1 c. quick-cooking oats	½ tsp. pepper
1 lb. lean ground beef	

Sauce:

½ brown sugar, packed	2 Tbsp. prepared mustard
2 tsp. lemon juice	14 oz. pasta sauce

1. Beat egg and milk together in a large bowl. Add rolled oats, onion, salt, and pepper. Stir.
2. Add ground beef; mix well. Shape into ¼ c. patties.
3. Cook in non-stick skillet, browning both sides, until no pink remains.
4. **For sauce:** heat and stir all 4 ingredients in saucepan until hot. Serve over patties.

Serves 6 with 2 patties each,
(or use 4, freezing the rest and serve with rice and corn or green beans)

Beefy Burritos

The perfect recipe for making lots for a crowd or lots for the freezer!

2 lbs. lean ground beef
1 onion, chopped
1 pkg. taco seasoning (3 Tbsp.)
¼ tsp. pepper
¾ c. taco sauce

Parsley to taste
1 c. sour cream
2 lbs. Monterey Jack cheese, grated
¼ tsp. oregano
flour tortillas

1. Brown ground beef with onions; pre-heat oven to 350° F.
2. Add taco seasoning, pepper, oregano, parsley, and sour cream.
3. Add ½ the cheese and ½ the taco sauce; mix well.
4. Place 2 to 3 Tbsp. of mixture on each tortilla, roll up and place seam side down in a 9" x 13" baking dish (sprayed with canola spray)
5. Top with remaining taco sauce and cheese; sprinkle with parsley and red pepper flakes, if you have them—makes for a festive look!
6. Bake for 25 min. (cover for 15 min. and uncover for the last 10 min.)

*Serves 16 with salsa, sour cream, and guacamole
(or use 4 and freeze the rest in dinner portions)*

The burritos are also nice with a salad or fresh veggies!

Cheddar Beef Tourtière

Very scrumptious! (and most great second time around!)

2 lb. ground beef	½ c. dark beer
2 carrots, sliced	1 onion, sliced
8 oz. sharp cheddar cheese, shredded	
2 stalks celery, sliced	Salt and pepper
1 clove, garlic, minced	1 baking potato, peeled/cubed

2 sheets frozen puffed pastry, thawed, but cold
1 large egg yolk, beaten with 1 Tbsp. water

1. Preheat oven to 375° F.
2. In a skillet, combine beef, carrots, onion, celery, garlic and potato; cook, breaking up the beef, over med. heat, until the beef is cooked through—about 15 min.
3. Lower the heat to medium, add the beer and cook for 10 min.
4. Add the cheese, 2 tsp. salt and ½ tsp. pepper—let cool.
5. On a floured surface, roll 1 puff pastry sheet into a 12" round. Place in a 10" skillet or deep pie dish. Roll the remaining sheet into an 11" round.
6. Using a slotted spoon, transfer the beef mixture to the pastry-lined skillet. Lightly brush the edge of the pastry with some of the egg wash.
7. Place the second pastry sheet on top of the beef mixture and press the edges of the pastry together to seal—trim to a ½" edge.
8. Place the tourtière on a baking sheet and brush the top with the remaining egg wash—cut an X or other design into the top of the pastry.
9. Sprinkle the tourtière with 1 tsp. salt and ½ tsp. pepper.
10. Bake for 45 min, tenting with foil if the pastry darkens before the time is up.
11. Transfer to a wire rack to rest for 15 min. before serving.

Serves 8 with salad and buns.

Cheesy Beef Burgers

Packed with flavour, these burgers!

1 lb. extra-lean ground beef	¼ c. BBQ sauce, divided
¼ c. cheese of choice, grated	4 burger buns
½ c. fresh bread crumbs	

1. Preheat BBQ to med-high heat.
2. Mix meat with cheese, bread crumbs, and 2 Tbsp. of BBQ sauce.
3. Shape mixture into 4 patties.
4. Place patties on the BBQ; cover with BBQ lid. Grill 4-6 min. on each side or until burgers are cooked through (160 F.), brushing with remaining 2 Tbsp. of BBQ sauce during the last 2 min. of grilling time.
5. Fill buns with burgers and fixings such as lettuce, tomato, onion, pickles……

Serves 4 with raw veggies

Coffee-Seasoned Steaks

Yes, really!

2 16 ox. Sirloin steaks
2 Tbsp. steak seasoning
1 Tbsp. chili powder
1 Tbsp. finely ground dark-roast coffee
1 Tbsp. canola oil
6 Tbsp. butter, cut into pieces
½ c. curly parsley, chopped fine

1. Heat a large cast iron skillet over high heat.
2. Rub the steaks with the steak seasoning, chili powder and coffee.
3. Add 1 Tbsp. oil to the skillet; turn the pan to coat evenly.
4. Add the steaks and cook, turning once, for 8 min.
5. Turn off the heat, tent with foil and let rest 10 min., turning once after 5 min.
6. Meanwhile, heat butter until foaming, in a small saucepan.
7. Stir in the parsley.
8. Slice the meat against the grain and divide into 4 portions. Pour the parsley butter over top.

Serve 4 with wild rice and salad, or sautéed small potatoes and asparagus.

Easier-than-Lasagna Burgers

Super Saturday Supper!

1 ½ lbs. ground beef, pork, and veal mix
Salt and pepper
2 Tbsp. extra-virgin olive oil
1 small onion, finely chopped
2 cloves garlic, minced
1 14.5 oz. can crushed Italian tomatoes
½ c. ricotta cheese
4 Kaiser or ciabatta rolls
Handful of basil leaves, torn
2 Tbsp. butter
2 Tbsp. flour
1 c. milk
Dash of nutmeg
¼ c. mozzarella, grated

1. In a large bowl, season the meat with salt and pepper.
2. Form into 4 patties, not too plump in the middle! (set aside)
3. In a saucepan, heat the olive oil, over medium heat.
4. Add the onion and cook until softened—about 5 min.
5. Add the garlic and cook for 2 more min.; stir in the tomatoes and season with salt and pepper.
6. Lower the heat and simmer for 5 min.; add the basil.
7. In a large skillet, heat a drizzle of olive oil over med-high heat; add the patties and cook until med-rare—7-8 min., turning once.
8. While the patties are cooking, in a small saucepan: melt the butter over med. heat, whisk in the flour for 1 min.; whisk in the milk; season with salt, pepper, and nutmeg; cook until thickened, about 5 min.
9. Stir in the ricotta and mozzarella.
10. Spoon some tomato sauce on the bottom half of the buns; top with the patties; spoon the cheese sauce on the patties and set the roll tops on the sauce.

Serves 4 with raw veggies and lots of napkins!

Having guests over? Add a Caesar salad!

Great Caesar Burgers

Makes a summer's eve' out of a snowy winter night!

1 ½ lb. lean ground beef	¼ tsp. pepper
¼ c. freshly grated parmesan cheese	2 Tbsp. extra virgin olive oil
2 Tbsp. lemon juice	1 garlic clove, minced
1 Tbsp. anchovy paste	4 Kaiser buns, halved
1 Tbsp. Worcestershire sauce	Romaine lettuce
1 egg, beaten	

1. Combine beef, 2 Tbsp. of the parmesan cheese, lemon juice, anchovy paste, Worcestershire sauce, egg and pepper.
2. Shape into 4 patties—¾" thick.
3. Broil or grill, until desired doneness.
4. Combine oil and garlic, brush over cut side of buns and grill/broil until toasted.
5. Sprinkle burgers with remaining cheese, place lettuce on bottom of each bun, top with burgers and bun tops—enjoy!

Serves 4 with raw veggies.

Make double the burgers and freeze half! (if freezing half the patties, start with fresh ground beef!)

Truly Divine Meatloaf

The perfect dinner for that snowy weekday night!

1 lb. lean ground beef	Salt and pepper to taste
1 med. onion, chopped	¼ c. ketchup
½ c. milk	¼ c. water
1 egg, beaten	1 tsp. dry mustard
8 crushed soda crackers	½ c. brown sugar

1. In a large bowl, combine ground beef, onion, milk, egg, crackers, salt and pepper; mix well.
2. Line an 8" x 4" x 3" loaf pan with plastic wrap and fill with the meat mixture.
3. Cover the top and place in the fridge overnight—this will firm up the mixture so it can be baked on a baking sheet, while holding its shape and reducing the amount of grease accumulation.
4. Before baking, turn out the meatloaf onto a foil-lined baking sheet. Make a groove down the centre of the surface of the loaf.
5. In a small bowl, combine ketchup, water, mustard, and brown sugar.
6. Pour ketchup mixture over the meatloaf and bake for 1 hour.
7. Slice ¾ to 1" wide to serve.

Serves 4 to 6 with mashed potatoes, green beans, and biscuits!

Freezes well or works great for meatloaf sandwiches!

Italian Beef and Ravioli Stew

So good on a drizzly day!

1 Tbsp. olive oil	1 med. onion, cut into wedges
2 lb. boneless chuck beef, cut into 1 inch pieces	
2 garlic cloves, minced	2 tsp. chopped fresh rosemary
2 cans (14.5 oz. ea.) tomatoes, chopped	
1 red pepper, cut into strips	1 tsp. ea. of balsamic vinegar, basil,
½ c. beef broth	1 tsp. olive oil
1 ½ c. frozen green beans	9 oz. cheese-filled ravioli

1. Heat oil in a 5 quart Dutch oven over med-high heat.
2. Cook onion, garlic, rosemary, and red pepper in oil for 5 min., stirring frequently, until onions are softened.
3. Stir in beef and cook for 8 min., stirring occasionally, until beef is lightly browned.
4. Stir in tomatoes and beef broth, with rosemary, balsamic vinegar and basil. Heat to boiling. Reduce heat to med-low. Cover and cook 50 min., stirring occasionally, until beef is tender.
5. Stir in frozen green beans and ravioli. Increase heat to med-high and cook 10 min., stirring occasionally, until ravioli is tender.

Serves 6 with crusty buns.

A wonderful use of leftover roast beef! Cut into 1 inch pieces; eliminate step 2. Add the beef after the tomatoes and beef broth have boiled in step 3. Reduce heat to low and simmer ½ hour to heat beef through. Go on to step 4.

Zesty Taco Pie

A taco dinner assembled in one dish!

1 lb. lean ground beef	3 eggs
½ c. onion, chopped	2 tomatoes, sliced
1 pkg. taco seasoning (3 Tbsp.)	1 c. cheddar cheese, grated
1-4oz. can green chilies, chopped	Salsa
	Shredded lettuce
1 ¼ c. milk	Sour cream
¾ c. biscuit mix	Guacamole

1. Brown ground beef with onion; preheat oven to 400 F, drain meat mixture and add taco seasoning.
2. Spread the mixture on the bottom of a 10" pie plate. Sprinkle with chilies.
3. In blender, beat milk, biscuit mix and eggs until smooth.
4. Pour over meat mixture.
5. Bake 25 min.
6. Top with tomato slices; sprinkle with grated cheese; bake 5 min. or until cheese is melted.
7. Cut into wedges and serve with salsa and other toppings.

Serves 6 with salad or raw veggies and dip.

Leftovers freeze well or love to go to lunch!

Chicken/Turkey

- Roast Herbed Chicken and Vegetables
- Southwestern Fajitas
- Almond-Dijon Baked Chicken
- BBQ Honey-Mustard Chicken Thighs
- Chicken Cordon Bleu, Made Easy
- Cozy-all-over Moroccan Chicken
- Fiesta-to-the-Max Chicken Enchiladas
- Fresh Veggie-Chicken BBQ Kebabs
- "In-a-Flash" Chicken Nacho-Style
- Mexican Chicken Dinner in a Pouch
- Scrumptious Chicken Thighs and Peppers
- Skillet Bruschetta Chicken
- Tortilla-Bake with Chicken and Spinach
- Yummy Chicken Skewers
- Cheesy-Apple Turkey Burgers
- Turkey-Barley Chowder with a Southern Flair
- Turkey-Mozza Burgers
- Spicy Pepper Jack Turkey Tortillas

Roast Herbed Chicken and Vegetables

Super way to start your Sun. AM with Sunday dinner set to cookin'!

3 Tbsp. olive or canola oil	½ tsp. salt
2 tsp. dried basil	¼ tsp. pepper
2 tsp. marjoram	1 tsp. rosemary
4 med. carrots, chopped into 1" pieces	
2 cloves garlic, minced	1 large onion, cut into wedges
3 lb. roasting chicken	6 potatoes, quartered

1. In a small bowl, combine oil, herbs, salt and pepper.
2. In shallow roasting pan, combine carrots and onion; drizzle half the oil mixture over the vegetables; toss to combine and push to the edges of the pan.
3. Place the chicken in the pan and brush the remaining oil mixture over the chicken.
4. Roast, uncovered, in a 325F oven for 2 hours, or until chicken is no longer pink inside and vegetables are tender.

Serves 6 with salad.

Southwestern Fajitas

A fun easy meal and makes great leftovers!

2 lbs. sirloin steak or 3 chicken breast halves (skinless, boneless)
Marinade for the meat:

½ c. canola oil	1 tsp. oregano
1/3 c. lime juice	Salt/pepper to taste
1/3 c. red wine vinegar (for steak only)	¼ tsp. cumin
1/3 c. chopped onion	2 garlic cloves, minced
1 tsp. sugar	

Toppings:

Onion slices, sautéed	Shredded lettuce (iceberg)
Green/red pepper strips, sautéed	Guacamole, sour cream, salsa

1. Combine marinade ingredients in a freezer bag.
2. Score both sides of the meat; add meat to marinade.
3. **Refrigerate meat for several hours; turn every few hrs.**
4. Remove meat from marinade and BBQ.
5. Slice meat into thin strips across the grain.
6. Wrap in warm tortillas with onions and peppers, with any of the additional toppings.

Serves 6 with salad on the side and taco chips!

Tip: wrap tortillas in foil package and place on the back shelf of the BBQ to warm up—really adds to the flavour.
Warmed up in the microwave is not quite the same!

Almond-Dijon Baked Chicken

Very easy to put together and sooooooooooo good!
Works well with any white fish as well.

4 small boneless skinless chicken breasts (or large, cut in half)
2 Tbsp. mayonnaise   2 Tbsp. Dijon mustard, crushed
6 whole grain crackers   1 Tbsp. flax seeds
¼ c. slivered almonds

1. Preheat oven to 375° F.
2. Place chicken on a parchment paper lined baking dish (or lightly grease with canola oil)
3. Mix mayonnaise and mustard until smooth.
4. Spread top-side of chicken with 1 Tbsp. of the mix.
5. Mix the crackers with almonds and flax seeds; sprinkle over the chicken, covering well.
6. Bake 20-25 min., making sure the chicken has reached 170 F.

Serves 4 with spinach salad and rice!

BBQ Honey-Mustard Chicken Thighs

Great way to jazz up those chicken thighs!

3 Tbsp. honey-mustard
2 Tbsp. canola oil
8 skinless, bone-in chicken thighs
2 limes—juice of one and other cut into 8 wedges
3 Tbsp. extra-virgin olive oil
2 Tbsp. chives, chopped

1. In a re-sealable bag, combine honey-mustard, oil and lime juice; add the chicken and let marinate at room temp. for 20 min.
2. Preheat the BBQ to med-high.
3. Add the chicken and cover the BBQ; cook for 10 min. on each side.
4. Serve the chicken with the lime wedges.

Serves 4 with 2 thighs each, sautéed potato wedges and Caesar salad.

Chicken Cordon Bleu, Made Easy

Goes together so well, anyone in the family can have this ready and in the oven for the rest of the family to come home to!

1 pkg. chicken stuffing mix	1 can cream of chicken soup
4 small chicken breasts	1 Tbsp. Dijon mustard
4 thin slices smoked ham	½ c. grated Swiss cheese (or mozzarella)

1. Preheat oven to 400 F.
2. Prepare stuffing as directed on package—set aside.
3. Place chicken in 13 X 9 inch baking dish; cover chicken with ham.
4. Mix soup and mustard; spoon over ham. Top with prepared stuffing.
5. Bake 25 min., or until chicken is cooked through (170 F.)
6. Sprinkle with cheese and bake an additional 5 min. or until cheese is melted.

Serves 4 with rice and salad, or asparagus.

Cozy-all-over Moroccan Chicken

A wonderfully exotic, but easy weekend dinner!

2 Tbsp. olive oil	¼ c. dried cranberries
1 ½ lbs. boneless, skinless, chicken breasts (allow 1 small per person)	
2 Tbsp. liquid honey	
½ c. onion, chopped	1 ½ tsp. cumin
1 garlic clove, minced	1 tsp. cinnamon
2 c. salsa	½ c. water
½ c. slivered almonds, toasted (or pecans)	

*** *almonds can be toasted in a baking dish, in oven, for a few minutes*

1. Preheat oven to 325F.
2. Heat oil in a large frying pan and brown the chicken.
3. Place chicken in the baking dish. (set aside the almonds first)
4. Lightly sauté the onions and garlic in the frying pan; spoon over the chicken.
5. In a bowl, combine the salsa, water, cranberries, honey, cumin, and cinnamon; pour over the chicken.
6. **Cover** and bake for 1 hour; sprinkle with the almonds.

Serves 4 with wild rice and salad or asparagus

Only 2 servings needed?
This is super for that second dinner or a treat for lunch

Fiesta-to-the-Max Chicken Enchiladas

Perfect use for the extra chicken breasts you BBQ'd last night or the roast chicken that is leftover!

1 ea. of onion and red pepper, chopped	1 Tbsp. cilantro, chopped
1 clove garlic, minced	1 tsp. ground cumin
4 cooked small chicken breasts,	1/c. grated tangy cheese, chopped
8 flour tortillas	1 c. salsa

125 g. light brick cream cheese, cubed Red pepper flakes
Parsley

1. Preheat oven to 350° F.
2. Heat large skillet, sprayed with cooking spray, to med. heat.
3. Add onions, peppers, and garlic; cook and stir 2 min.
4. Add chicken, ¼ c. salsa, cream cheese, cilantro and cumin; mix well. Cook until heated through, stirring occasionally.
5. Add ¼ c. of the grated cheese; mix well.
6. Place about 1/3 c. of the chicken mixture onto each tortilla and roll up.
7. Place tortillas, seam side down in a 13 X 9 inch baking dish, sprayed with cooking spray; top with remaining salsa and grated cheese. Sprinkle with red pepper flakes and parsley.
8. Cover with foil, tenting over cheese. Bake 20 min.
9. Remove foil and bake 10 min. more.

Serves 4—8, depending on how many enchiladas everyone has!

Add a salad to the "fiesta" and serve sour cream with guacamole, on the side, for the enchiladas.

The above method is great for leftover stir fries, as well. If any of the enchiladas are leftover (IF!), they are great for lunches!

Fresh Veggie-Chicken BBQ Kebabs

Colourful and healthy chicken with veggies sweetened up with pineapple— most festive for a summer's eve!

½ c. BBQ sauce
2 c. 1 ½" fresh pineapple chunks
1 lb. chicken breasts, cut into 1 ½" pieces
3 Tbsp. frozen orange juice concentrate, thawed
1 ea. red and green pepper, cut into 1 ½" pieces

1. Preheat grill to med. high heat.
2. Prepare 4 kebabs with 2 wooden skewers each (this prevents the pieces from spinning when turned during BBQing) Alternate the chicken with the peppers and pineapple.
3. Mix BBQ sauce with the juice concentrate; brush some of the sauce onto the kebabs.
4. Grill 8 to 10 min., or until chicken is cooked through, turning and brushing occasionally with the remaining sauce.

Serves 4 with rice and salad. (Spinach or Caesar for example)

If you prefer, 8 kebabs can be made with the meat, peppers and pineapple not as packed onto the skewers—although it is easier to manage 4 kebabs rather than 8 on the BBQ! These can also be done under the broiler on a rainy day, or mid-winter!

"In-a-Flash" Chicken Nacho-Style

This goes together so quick—great for a weekday meal or a fun, relaxing Sat. Supper!

4 small chicken breasts
½ c. chunky salsa
¼ c. sour cream
½ c. crushed tortilla chips
½ c. "Tex-Mex" style cheese, grated

1. Pre-heat oven to 400 F.
2. Place chicken on foil-lined baking sheet.
3. Slice 3 cuts into the top of each chicken breast.
4. Top each chicken breast evenly with salsa, sour cream, and tortilla chips.
5. Bake 20 min. Remove from oven and sprinkle with the cheese.
6. Bake an additional 10 min., or until chicken is cooked through—170 F. internal temp.

Serves 4 with rice or noodles and broccoli or salad.

Mexican Chicken Dinner in a Pouch

SO quick and easy to dash together—for mid-week or for guests on Saturday night!

4 small chicken breasts, skinless, boneless
4 tsp. taco seasoning   ½ c. salsa
½ lb. red potatoes, thinly sliced, not peeled
½ c. cheddar cheese, grated   ¼ c. sour cream

1. Preheat oven to 400 F.
2. Sprinkle chicken with seasoning mix.
3. Place ½ c. of potatoes in the centre of each of 4 large pieces of heavy foil; place chicken, salsa, and cheese on top of the potatoes.
4. Bring up foil sides—double-fold top and ends, leaving room for heat circulation inside.
5. Place pouches on a large baking sheet.
6. Bake 30—35 min., or until chicken is cooked through (170 F.)
7. Remove pouches from the oven and let rest 5 min. before opening—cut slits in the foil to release steam. Serve with sour cream.

Serves 4—just add asparagus or salad!

Scrumptious Chicken Thighs and Peppers

A great roasted dinner in one dish—so easy, so good!

8 chicken thighs	1 green pepper, cut into strips
4-6 garlic cloves, halved	1 onion, cut into wedges
3-4 new potatoes, quartered	½ tsp. dried thyme
1 red pepper, cut into strips	Salt and pepper, to taste
Fresh mushrooms, halved	1-2 Tbsp. olive oil

1. Preheat oven to 425F.
2. In a 9" x 13" baking dish, lightly coat with canola spray.
3. Toss all ingredients with olive oil and spread in a single layer in the pan, with chicken upside down.
4. Roast, uncovered, until vegetables are tender-crisp, about 30 min.
5. Turn chicken and vegetables; cook until chicken is no longer pink in the center—15-20 min. longer.
6. Arrange on a heated platter and serve immediately.

Serves 4 with small chicken thighs or 8 with large chicken thighs!

This dinner is complete by itself or you could add a salad.

Skillet Bruschetta Chicken

Very quick to prepare and cook—an elegant dinner even for a weeknight! (or at least a Friday night!)

2 Tbsp. sundried tomato and oregano salad dressing	1 large tomato, chopped
	1 red pepper, chopped
4 small boneless chicken breasts, halved	2 cloves garlic, minced
1 ½ c. instant rice, uncooked	½ c. mozzarella cheese, grated
1 can (19 oz.) Italian-style diced tomatoes, drained	
3 Tbsp. fresh basil, chopped	

1. Heat dressing in a large skillet on med. heat.
2. Add chicken, peppers, and garlic, cover.
3. Cook 10 min. or until chicken is cooked through (170F), stirring occasionally and turning chicken after 5 min.
4. Remove chicken from skillet—cover to keep warm.
5. To skillet, add canned tomatoes, **1 c.** of chopped tomatoes, and rice—bring to a boil.
6. Reduce heat to low, simmer, uncovered, for 10 min.
7. Meanwhile, combine cheese with the basil and remaining chopped tomatoes.
8. Return chicken to the skillet and sprinkle with the cheese mixture. Cover and cook 5 min. or until chicken is heated through and cheese is melted.

Serves 4 with spinach salad—enjoy!

This recipe can easily be doubled to include guests or to freeze half for a great meal next month!

Tortilla-Bake with Chicken and Spinach

Pop this in the oven and make a salad!

1 Tbsp. extra-virgin olive oil
4 small chicken breasts
½ red onion, sliced thinly
3 c. baby spinach
2 c. pepper jack cheese, shredded

4 large flour tortillas cut into wedges
Salt and pepper
1 ½ c. salsa
¾ c. ricotta cheese

1. Preheat oven to 450 F.
2. In a large skillet, heat the olive oil over med-high heat.
3. Season the chicken with salt and pepper; add to the pan and cook, turning once, until cooked through—about 5 min.
4. Let meat cool and then shred the meat.
5. Whisk the salsa and ricotta together with salt and pepper—dash of each.
6. In a greased 9-inch square baking dish, layer 1/3 of the salsa mixture, tortillas, chicken, onion, spinach, and pepper jack cheese; repeat twice more.
7. Bake until golden brown—15-20 min.
8. Let stand 10 min. before serving.

Serves 4 with sour cream and guacamole for garnish; salad or raw veggies on the side

---

This is a great use of cooked chicken (ie from a roast) or cooked ground beef from making tacos!

Yummy Chicken Skewers

Wonderful with that Naan Bread on Saturday eve'!

Marinade: (chicken will be marinated overnight)

3 garlic cloves, crushed	2 tsp. Dijon mustard
2 Tbsp. honey	2 tsp. tobacco sauce
¼ c. ketchup	Salt and pepper to taste

3 large boneless, skinless chicken breasts, cut into thin strips
12   10" wooden skewers

1. Soak skewers in water at least ½ hour.
2. For **marinade:** combine all ingredients and add chicken; toss until covered.
3. Place chicken in a non-metallic dish and cover to marinate **overnight**.
4. Preheat broiler to high.
5. Thread chicken onto skewers and arrange over wire racks on a foil-lined baking sheet.
6. Bake for 6—7 min., turning occasionally, until well-browned and cooked through. (on the **BBQ** these take 5—6 min.)

Serves 6—8 with Naan bread and Greek or Spinach salad.

Leftovers (if any!) make for a super meal on a busy week night

Cheesy-Apple Turkey Burgers

These are SO good!

2 lbs. ground turkey breast	1 apple, cut into 12 slices
4 scallions, finely chopped	4 sharp cheddar cheese slices
1/3 c. fresh parsley, chopped	1 Tbsp. BBQ seasoning
1/4 c. whole-berry cranberry sauce	1 tsp. poultry seasoning
2 Tbsp. extra-virgin olive oil	2 Tbsp. grainy mustard
4 sandwich-size English muffins, halved and toasted	4 leaves red/green leaf lettuce

1. In a large bowl combine the turkey, scallions, parsley, BBQ seasoning, and poultry seasoning.
2. Form mixture into 4 patties.
3. In a large skillet, heat the olive oil over med-high heat. Add the patties and cook for 6 min. on each side.
4. Top each with 2-3 apple slices and 1 cheese slice. Cover.
5. Cook until the cheese melts—1-2 min.
6. In a small bowl, mix together the grainy mustard and cranberry sauce; spread on muffin tops.
7. Place the lettuce leaves on the muffin bottoms, followed by the patties and the muffin tops.

Serves 4 with raw veggies

These burgers can also be done on the BBQ and Kaiser buns can be used in place of the English muffins.

Turkey-Barley Chowder with a Southern Flair

Another superb use of that Christmas Turkey!

5 c. turkey stock (or chicken broth)	1 bunch scallions, sliced thinly
¾ c. pearl barley	1 ½ c. tomato sauce
2 ½ c. cooked turkey, chopped	1 green pepper, diced
1 ½ c. asparagus, cut into 1 ½" pieces	1 lb. large shrimp, peeled and deveined
2 tsp. hot sauce	Sour cream for serving

1. In a small saucepan, bring 2 c. turkey stock and the barley to a boil. Lower the heat, cover and simmer until tender—about 40 min.
2. In a large saucepan, bring the remaining 3 c. of stock, tomato sauce, green pepper, and cooked barley to a boil.
3. Stir in the asparagus and scallions, lower the heat and simmer for 10 min.
4. Add the turkey and shrimp; cook until the shrimp is opaque—about 3 min.—stir in the hot sauce.

Serves 6 with sour cream and buns

Alternate for the asparagus—green beans or broccoli

Turkey-Mozza Burgers

Scrumptious use of that holiday turkey!

4 Tbsp. butter	½ c. parsley, chopped
1 small Macintosh apple, finely chopped	2 Tbsp. Dijon mustard
1 small onion, finely chopped	2 tsp. poultry seasoning
1 small rib of celery, finely chopped	4 Mozzarella slices
Salt and pepper	1/3 c. whole-berry cranberry sauce
½ c. breadcrumbs	3 Tbsp. sour cream
1 lb. dark turkey meat, ground	2 Tbsp. chives, chopped
1 large egg	4 large sourdough English muffins
Extra-virgin olive oil	4 thin slices red onion
4 leaves red-leaf lettuce	

1. Heat a large skillet over med. heat. Add the butter to melt, then add the apple, onion, and celery; season with salt and pepper.
2. Cover and cook until softened—3 to 4 min. Stir in the breadcrumbs, then transfer to a bowl to cool; reserve the skillet.
3. In the bowl, mix in the turkey, egg, mustard, and poultry seasoning; season with salt and pepper.
4. Form the turkey mixture into four 4" patties.
5. Wipe out the reserved skillet and add 1Tbsp. olive oil. Warm over med-high heat, add the patties and cook, turning once, until cooked through—8 to 10 min.
6. Top with the mozzarella during the last minute.
7. Meanwhile, in a small bowl, mix the cranberry sauce, sour cream, and chives.
8. Serve the patties on the English muffins with the onion slices, lettuce and cranberry-sour cream sauce.

Serves 4, with veggies and dip

Spicy Pepper Jack Turkey Tortillas

A very "cool" Saturday supper—heat 'em up for a busy Monday! (Another use of leftover turkey ......)

6 Tortillas
3 Tbsp. extra-virgin olive oil
2 onions, sliced thinly
Salt and pepper
8 oz. pepper jack cheese, grated

1/3 c. mayonnaise
2 c. cooked turkey meat, shredded
1 c. baby spinach
Lemon wedges, for serving

1. Place rack in the lower half of the oven and preheat to 450 F.
2. In a large skillet, heat 1 Tbsp. of the olive oil over med. heat.
3. Add the onions, season with salt and pepper, and cook, stirring occasionally, until soft and golden—about 12 min.
4. Brush each tortilla with 1 tsp. olive oil and place on parchment paper.
5. Place the tortillas, with the parchment paper, on baking sheets; bake until slightly browned—2 min.; transfer to a rack to cool.
6. In a medium bowl, stir together the cheese and mayonnaise, spread on the tortillas and scatter the onions on top.
7. Bake until the cheese is melted and bubbly—about 2 min.
8. Top each tortilla with the turkey and spinach; drizzle with olive oil and season with salt and pepper.
9. Fold in half and serve with lemon wedges.

Serves 6 with raw veggies and dip.

Pork

Cranberry–Orange Pork Chops on the Slow Side

Fall for Pork and Apples

Ginger Pork Stir-Fry

Glazed-over Apricot Pork

Grilled Pineapple-Pork Skewers

Mushroom Pork Stew

Pork and Peppers Stir-Fry

Pork Chops on Bed of Corn Bread Stuffing and Broccoli Mix

Stuffed and Wrapped Pork Chops

All Cheesy Ham and Eggs

Ham and Cheese Frittata

So Good Spiced Ham Slices

Fiesta Peppered Sausage Burritos

Cranberry–Orange Pork Chops on the S*low* Side

A super tender treatment of pork chops!

2 c. carrots, coarsely chopped
8 boneless pork loin chops, cut ¾" thick
1 12 oz. jar cranberry-orange sauce
2 Tbsp. quick-cooking tapioca
Small can of apricots, sliced

1 tsp. lemon peel, finely shredded
½ tsp. cardamom

4 c. hot-cooked rice

1. Place carrots in a 3.5-4 quart slow cooker.
2. Place pork chops on carrots.
3. Combine cranberry-orange sauce, tapioca, lemon peel, and cardamom; place over meat.
4. Cover; cook on low-heat for 7-8 hrs. (or high heat for 3.5-4 hrs.)
5. Add apricots to pork mixture; turn off **s*low* cooker**.
6. Cover; let stand for 5 min.

Serves 8 over cooked rice, with asparagus or green beans on the side.

Fall for Pork and Apples

A great looking dish for an Autumn Sunday!

2 c. uncooked broad noodles	1 can cream of celery soup
½ c. apple juice	2 Tbsp. canola oil
1 Tbsp. fresh thyme, chopped	¼ tsp. ground cinnamon
1 lb. pork tenderloin, cut into ¼" slices	¼ tsp. pepper
2 c. mushrooms, sliced	1 red apple, unpeeled, sliced
½ c. onion, chopped	

1. Preheat oven to 350° F.
2. Cook noodles, as usual.
3. Heat 1 Tbsp. canola oil on med. high; cook pork until browned and cooked through—about 4 min. per side.
4. Reduce heat to medium and add mushrooms, with onion; cook about 5 min.
5. Mix soup, juice, thyme, cinnamon, and pepper in shallow 2 qt. baking dish. (prep first with canola spray) Stir in noodles and mushroom mixture.
6. Place the pork on the noodle mixture with the apple slices.
7. Bake at 350° F for 30 min.

Serves 4 with a salad.

Freeze leftovers —works well heated up – 40 min. @ 325F)

Ginger Pork Stir-Fry

Elegant Saturday night dinner—for family and guests!

1 Tbsp. canola oil	1 Tbsp. ketchup
½ onion, chopped	¼ tsp. ginger
½ green pepper, sliced	1 garlic clove, minced
1 carrot, grated	2 tsp. cornstarch
3 Tbsp. white vinegar	1 Tbsp. water
¼ c. brown sugar, packed	1 Tbsp. canola oil
1 Tbsp. soy sauce	

1 lb. boneless pork loin, cut into thin strips, trimmed of fat

1. **For ginger sauce:** Heat canola oil in skillet. Add onion, green pepper, and carrot; stir-fry until soft.
2. Add next 6 ingredients and stir.
3. Mix cornstarch with water in small bowl; add to sauce; stir until thickened. **Keep warm.**
4. Heat 2nd amount of canola oil in separate skillet; **add pork strips** and stir fry until no longer pink.
5. Add sauce and stir.

Serves 4 over rice. Tackle with chopsticks, if you can!

Chicken or sirloin can be used in place of the pork; chopped asparagus, broccoli, and/or red pepper can also be used for the veggies ; you can also throw in some cashews at the end!

Glazed-over Apricot Pork

Great to have cooking on a busy—or relaxing—Sunday!

1   3 to 3 ½ lb. boneless, pork shoulder roast
1   18 oz. jar apricot jam   1 large onion, chopped
¼ c. chicken broth   2 tbsp. Dijon-type mustard

1. Trim fat from roast; if needed, cut to fit slow cooker and place in slow cooker.
2. Combine jam, broth, mustard, and onions; pour over meat.
3. Cover and cook on low heat for 10-12 hours (high for 3-6 hours)
4. Transfer meat to serving platter; skim fat from the sauce and spoon some over the meat.

Serves 8 (or 4 with leftovers!)

Changes: other jams could be used, such as peach, apple jelly, blueberry, pomegranate, marmalade

Grilled Pineapple-Pork Skewers

Give your summer BBQ a tropical flare with these easy kebabs!

1 20 oz. can pineapple chunks, drained with juice reserved
1 clove garlic, minced   Salt and pepper
2 Tbsp. soy sauce   2 Tbsp. fresh ginger, finely grated
1 ½ lb. pork loin, cut into 1 inch cubes
2 Tbsp. canola oil

1. In a re-sealable plastic bag, combine the pineapple juice, garlic, and oil; season with salt and pepper.
2. Add the pork and let marinate for 30 min., at room temp.
3. Preheat an outdoor grill to med-high.
4. Thread the marinated pork and pineapple chunks onto 4 10-inch skewers.
5. Grill the kebabs, turning occasionally, until golden and cooked through, about 10-12 min.

Serves 4 with wild rice and salad (Spinach, Caesar or Coleslaw) Recipe easily doubles for more guests!

Mushroom Pork Stew

Such a nice, comforting dish to have on a cool, rainy night!

1 Tbsp. canola oil	1 ½ c. frozen pearl onions
1 Tbsp. margarine	2 garlic cloves, minced
3 med. carrots, sliced diagonally	1 c. fresh mushrooms, sliced
1 small onion, stuffed with 4 whole cloves	1 tsp. salt
1 ½ lb. pork loin, cut into 1 inch pieces	2 ½ c. chicken broth
1/8 tsp. pepper	1 c. white wine (or chicken broth)
1 c. whipping (heavy) cream	Chopped fresh parsley
1/3 c. flour	

1. Heat oil and margarine in a 5 quart Dutch oven over med-high heat.
2. Cook garlic and mushrooms in the oil mixture for 6 min., stirring frequently, until mushrooms are softened.
3. Stir in pork and cook for 7 min., stirring frequently, until browned.
4. Add broth, wine, pearl onions, carrots, onion with cloves, salt and pepper. Heat to boiling; reduce heat to med-low.
5. Cover and cook 30 min., stirring occasionally, until pork is tender and no longer pink in the center.
6. Remove onion with cloves; discard. Beat in whipping cream and flour with wire whisk. Cook 6 more min., stirring constantly, until hot and slightly thickened.
7. Sprinkle with parsley.

Serves 6 with crusty rolls.

A great use of the leftover pork roast from Sunday— add pork pieces in step 4 to heat through.

Pork and Peppers Stir-Fry

So colourful! Do the cutting the night before and it is a quick stir fry on your busy week night

1 lb. boneless pork loin	3 Tbsp. cornstarch
3 Tbsp. canola oil	1 c. chicken broth
1 of each—red/green/yellow peppers, cut into 1" pieces	
3 sprigs green onions, cut into 1" pieces	½ c. teriyaki sauce
4 cloves garlic, minced	

1. Cut the pork into ¼ inch-thick slices, then into ¼" wide pieces.
2. Toss pork with 2 Tbsp. cornstarch.
3. In a large skillet, heat 1½ Tbsp. oil over med-high heat. Add the garlic, cook 2 min.; add the pork and cook for 2 min., until no longer pink. Transfer to a bowl.
4. Add the remaining 1½ Tbsp. oil to the skillet and cook the peppers until crisp-tender—about 2 min.
5. In a small bowl, stir together the chicken broth, teriyaki sauce and remaining 1 Tbsp. cornstarch; pour over the peppers and cook, stirring, until the sauce is thickened—1-2 min.
6. Return the pork mixture to the skillet, add the green onions and stir until heated through—1-2 min.

Serves 4 with rice.

Chicken or beef can easily be substituted for the pork; if using beef, use beef broth instead of the chicken broth. Sliced mushrooms can also be added —cook with the meat.

Pork Chops on Bed of Corn Bread Stuffing and Broccoli Mix

So nice to have this dinner cooking away in the oven while you prepare a salad! Perfect for a Saturday meal—even Sunday!

4 pork rib chops   ¼ c. butter, melted
1 10 oz. can golden mushroom condensed soup
1 16 oz pkg. frozen broccoli, cauliflower and carrots
½ of a 16 oz. pkg. of corn bread stuffing mix (or 3 c.)

1. Pre-heat the oven to 350° F. Lightly spray a 13"x 9" casserole dish, and a large skillet, with cooking spray.
2. Brown the chops, on med. high heat, in the skillet. Remove chops from the skillet and set aside.
3. In a large bowl, combine the soup and melted butter. Stir in the frozen vegetables and stuffing mix; spread on the bottom of the casserole dish.
4. Place the chops on the stuffing mixture.
5. Cover and bake for 1 hour.

Serves 4 with a salad.

This can also be made in the slow cooker, same procedure, and cook for 5 to 6 hours on low-setting.

Stuffed and Wrapped Pork Chops

WOW! This is so good for a quick end-of-the-week meal or an elegant dinner for guests Sat. eve' or impressive Sun. Family dinner!

4 Bone-in Pork Chops
½ c. bread crumbs
2 Tbsp. dried cranberries
(or dried apricots or diced apple)
4 slices Prosciutto
Salt & Pepper to taste
2 Tbsp. olive oil

1. In small bowl, mix bread crumbs and cranberries.
2. Slice pork chops open around the tenderloin, leaving one side intact; slice down ¼".
3. Peel back top layer of opening to form a pocket.
4. Stuff this area with the bread crumb mixture.
5. Wrap one piece of prosciutto over the pocket and secure with toothpicks.
6. Heat olive oil to med. high in pan large enough for the pork chops.
7. Pre-heat oven to 350° F.
8. Sprinkle each side of the pork chops with salt & pepper before cooking that side.
9. Cook each side of the pork chops to golden, about 10-15 min. a side.
10. Place pork chops in a small roasting pan sprayed with Canola spray.
11. Bake uncovered for 15 min.
12. Cover and bake for 30 min. more.

Serves 4 with applesauce, wild rice and spinach salad or coleslaw.

All Cheesy Ham and Eggs

Great for brunch or an easy supper.

6 slices white bread, crusts removed
8 oz. sliced deli ham
3 c. Monterey cheese, grated
3 Tbsp. finely chopped chives

6 large eggs
8 Tbsp. milk
Salt and pepper
2 plum tomatoes, thinly sliced

1. Preheat oven to 350° F. **Grease** a 2 qt. casserole dish.
2. Layer the bread, ham, 2 c. of cheese and 2 Tbsp. chives in the dish.
3. In a medium bowl, whisk the eggs, milk, dash of salt and dash of pepper.
4. Pour into the dish and top with the tomato slices.
5. Bake the dish until the eggs are evenly set, about 30 min.
6. Sprinkle the remaining cheese and chives on top and bake until golden.

Serves 6 with biscuits and salad, or raw veggies and dip.

Ham and Cheese Frittata

Quick way to use that leftover ham—quick to prepare and quick to eat! Works well for a zippy week-day meal or relaxing Sat. Brunch!

1 ½ c. cheddar cheese, grated   ½ c. sliced mushrooms
1/2 c. diced ham   6 eggs, well beaten
1/3 c. peppers, diced (whatever colours you like!)
¼ c. milk   1 Tbsp. parsley

1. Pre-heat oven to 350° F.
2. Spray a 9" glass pie-plate with Canola spray.
3. Sprinkle ham, cheese, peppers, and mushrooms on the surface of the pie plate. (save 1/4 c. cheese for the last 10 min.)
4. Beat the eggs with the milk until frothy.
5. Pour the egg mixture over the ham mixture.
6. Bake for 20 min. until starting to look set on the surface and slightly golden.
7. Sprinkle on the reserved cheese with parsley.
8. Bake for 10 min. more.
9. Slice into wedges.

*Serves 6 with sausages and fruit or coleslaw.
Leftovers freeze well to be used later as another quick meal!*

So Good Spiced Ham Slices

A super easy use of ham saved from Sunday's dinner!

¼ c. brown sugar
¼ tsp. allspice
12 slices ham, 1 cm thick

14 oz. crushed pineapple with juice
1/8 tsp. cloves

1. Preheat oven to 400 F.
2. Combine first 4 ingredients in a bowl.
3. Place ham slices in a single layer on a *ungreased* baking sheet with sides.
4. Spoon pineapple mixture over ham.
5. Bake for 40 min., **uncovered**.

Serves 6 (2 slices each) with sautéed potatoes and green beans.

Fiesta Peppered Sausage Burritos

Great for brunch, lunch, or casual supper

½ red onion, thinly sliced
Salt and pepper
Extra virgin olive oil
1 each of red and green pepper, chopped
1 c. salsa
6 large eggs, beaten
1 c. pepper jack cheese, grated
1/3 lb. Farmer's sausage, chopped
4 large tortillas, warmed
Guacamole and sour cream

1. Heat 1 Tbsp. olive oil over medium-high heat. Add the sausage and cook until browned, 3-4 min.
2. Add the peppers and onion, season with salt and pepper; cook 5 min. more.
3. In separate skillet, heat 1 Tbsp. olive oil over medium heat. Add the eggs, season with salt and pepper; scramble just until the "gloss" is gone, 2-3 min.
4. Divide the scramble eggs among the tortillas and serve the sausage mixture on top.
5. Roll up as for a taco and eat with your hands (good "grab and go" breakfast/lunch) or roll up to eat with knife and fork at brunch, or supper!

Serves 4 with salsa, sour cream and guacamole for dipping.

For breakfast, brunch, or lunch a fruit salad is nice on the side or serve with a spinach salad at supper.

Fish/Seafood

Almond-Encrusted Tilapia

Clammed-up Chowder

Fishy Tomato Soup

Grilled Salmon

Ola! Crab Enchiladas

SO Cool Crab Cakes

Wild Rice Stuffed Salmon

Almond-Encrusted Tilapia

Prep the night before and all it takes is 25 min. of baking on a busy weeknight; it is most presentable for a Sunday dinner as well!

2 ¼ lbs. Tilapia (or other whitefish) fillets

1 tsp. pepper	2 tsp. chives, chopped
1 Tbsp. onion flakes	1/8 tsp. paprika
½ tsp. salt	½ c. sliced almonds, toasted
3 Tbsp. lemon juice	Lemon wedges

Sauce:

½ Tbsp. cornstarch

1 Tbsp. water

1. Preheat oven to 400 F.
2. Sprinkle fish fillets with lemon juice. Lay ½ of fillets in 13" X 9" pan, sprayed with canola spray.
3. Sprinkle with next four ingredients. Top with remaining fillets.
4. Sprinkle with paprika and almonds
5. Bake 25 min., or until fish flakes easily with a fork.
6. For sauce, remove liquid from pan to a small saucepan with a turkey baster. Combine cornstarch and water in a small cup, and then add to the liquid. Heat, stirring constantly, until boiling and thickened. Makes 1 cup of sauce—serve over fish.

Serves 6-8 with wild rice and asparagus. (great with those lemon wedges!)

Clammed-up Chowder

A super comfort soup on those chilly nights!

6 Tbsp. butter or margarine	1 large potato, sliced
1 large onion, chopped	1 tin large butter clams
1 large carrot, grated	2 tins baby clams, with juice
1 large celery stalk, grated	1 c. light cream
2 Tbsp. chopped parsley	½ tsp. salt
2 c. flour	½ tsp. pepper
4 c. milk	¼ tsp. paprika
1 small tin evaporated milk	1 tsp. seafood seasoning

1. Melt the margarine in a large Dutch oven.
2. Saute the onion, carrot, celery, and parsley until the onion is soft—not brown.
3. Stir in the flour. Gradually add the milk and evaporated milk, stirring constantly.
4. Cook until the mixture thickens.
5. Peel and dice the potato and cook in a small pot with the juice of the large clams.
6. When the potato is soft, add it to the vegetable mixture, including the clam juice.
7. Chop the large clams coarsely and add to the above with the baby clams.
8. Stir in the cream; add the salt and pepper and heat, but do not boil.
9. Saute the paprika and seafood seasoning in a little margarine and add at the last minute. Do not stir—this will float on the top for a garnish.

Serves 10-12 with biscuits and salad (or 4 with 2 batches to freeze!)

A lot of steps, but worth it—this soup is SO good!

Fishy Tomato Soup

Nothing's "fishy" about this soup—it is so good on a cold snowy day! (Also good on an active summer day spent on the water!)

1 Tbsp. olive oil	1 tsp. finely chopped garlic
2 cans (14 oz. ea.) Italian-style tomatoes	2 med. stalks celery, chopped
2 cans (14 oz. ea.) chicken broth	1 med. onion, chopped
1 c. dry white wine (or vegetable broth)	1 ½ tsp. salt
1 ½ lb. assorted white fish fillets, cut into 1" pieces	
1 tbsp. fresh parsley, chopped	½ tsp. pepper
1 bay leaf	Grated lemon peel

1. Heat oil in 5-6 quart Dutch oven over med. heat.
2. Cook garlic, celery, onion, parsley, and bay leaf in oil 5-6 min., stirring frequently, until celery is crisp-tender.
3. Stir in tomatoes, broth and wine. Heat to boiling, over high heat; reduce heat to med-low.
4. Cover and simmer 20 min., stirring occasionally.
5. Stir in fish, salt, and pepper. Cover and simmer 8-10 min. or until fish flakes easily with a fork. Remove bay leaf.
6. Top soup with lemon peel.

Serves 8—10 with crusty buns.

Grilled Salmon

A fun and quick topping for Salmon!

1 untreated cedar plank   1/4 c. fresh parsley, chopped fine
½ c. oil-packed sun-dried tomatoes, drained and chopped fine
1 lb. salmon fillet, 1 inch thick
½ c. sundried tomato and oregano dressing

1. Set plank in water, weighed down to be covered. Soak for 4 hrs. or overnight.
2. Pre-heat BBQ to medium heat. Mix dressing, parsley, and tomatoes; set aside.
3. Brush top of cedar plank with 1 Tbsp. oil, top with fish.
4. Place fish on BBQ and grill 10 min.
5. Brush with dressing mixture; continue to grill for 10 more min. or until fish flakes easily with a fork.

Serves 8 with wild rice and Spinach Salad

The salmon could be done in the oven @ 400 F. for 20 min.—place fish on parchment paper-lined baking sheet.

Other fish, such as tilapia or steelhead trout could be used instead of the salmon

Ola! Crab Enchiladas

*A fun dish for Saturday night—freezes well for a weeknight dinner also—**bonus!***

1 Tbsp. hard margarine	¼ tsp. dried basil
1 c. onion, chopped	¼ tsp. salt
14 oz. canned tomatoes, chopped	1/8 tsp. seasoning salt
7 ½ oz. tomato sauce	1 lb. crabmeat
4 oz. canned jalapenos, chopped	1 ½ c. Monterey cheese, grated
1 tsp. sugar	½ tsp. dried oregano
12 corn tortillas	

1. Preheat oven to 350° F.
2. Melt margarine in skillet; add onion and sauté until soft.
3. Combine next 8 ingredients in saucepan; mix well and add the onion. Bring to a boil, stirring often; simmer, **uncovered**, for 10 min.
4. Spray a 9 X 13 inch pan with canola spray and spread on ¼ c. of the sauce; set pan aside and reserve ½ c. of the sauce.
5. Stir crabmeat, ½ c. of the cheese, and reserved sauce in a bowl.
6. Spread remaining sauce lightly onto each tortilla. Place ¼ c. of the crab mixture onto the end of each tortilla and roll up.
7. Place tortillas seam side down in prepared pan. Spread remaining sauce over tortillas.
8. Sprinkle remaining cheese over the tortillas and bake, **uncovered**, for 25 min.

Serves 12 with 1 tortilla each, or serve 4 and freeze the rest!

Goes well with spinach salad or fresh veggies. Added garnish: parsley, basil and/or chilli flakes with sour cream served on the side. Guacamole is also nice!

Salmon or tuna can be used in place of the crab.

SO Cool Crab Cakes

A super supper to get on the table in a flash during the week!

½ lb. crab (fresh, frozen, OR canned!) 1 Tbsp. grainy mustard
1 c. **fresh** bread crumbs 1 green onion, finely chopped
1 large egg Salt and freshly ground pepper, dash ea.
½ c. Panko crumbs (or dry crumbs) 2 Tbsp. canola oil

1. Combine crab, bread crumbs, egg, mustard, green onion, salt and pepper in a medium bowl.
2. Fill a shallow bowl or pie plate with Panko, or dry bread crumbs.
3. Shape the crab mixture into small patties and coat with the Panko crumbs.
4. Place canola oil into a large, heavy skillet, set over med-high heat.
5. Cook the patties until golden, about 5 min. per side (flip carefully!)

Serves 4—2 patties each, with wild rice and spinach salad, or asparagus

> Smaller patties could be used as an appetizer!

Wild Rice Stuffed Salmon

SO easy and so elegant!

1 whole salmon (or trout or any other whole fish)

Pepper	Garlic Powder
Seasoning salt	Parsley
Basil	sprinkling of each seasoning

1 package wild rice mix (any flavour of your choice—make enough for 4 servings)

1 green pepper, chopped   1 onion, chopped

1 c. fresh mushrooms, sliced

1. Preheat oven to 325F. Prepare a baking sheet with parchment paper.
2. Cook rice according to package instructions.
3. Saute vegetables in small amount of olive oil.
4. Add rice to onion mixture and stir.
5. Place the whole fish on the parchment paper; sprinkle seasonings inside and outside the salmon; rub to spread all over.
6. Stuff the fish with the rice mixture. If there is any left over, fill a small casserole and put in the oven with the fish.
7. Cook the fish for 35-40 min.

Serves 4 with asparagus

Rice & Pasta

The Best Macaroni and Cheese

Cheesy Broccoli Rice Bake

Wild Rice Soup

THE BEST Macaroni and Cheese!

This goes back to my grandmother's day, when every Thursday night was macaroni night and my Great-Uncle Gordon always "happened" to drop by!

2 c. macaroni	3 c. boiling water
1 Tbsp. canola oil	2 tsp. salt

1. Preheat oven to 350° F
2. In a large, uncovered saucepan, cook the macaroni in boiling water, canola oil and salt until tender (about 5-7 min.)

For white sauce:

3 Tbsp. flour	3 Tbsp. margarine
Sprinkle salt and pepper	2 c. milk with 4 Tbsp.
Sprinkle paprika	2 c. grated cheddar cheese

3. Saute flour and margarine together; stir in the salt, pepper, milk, and cheese until mixture boils, thickens, and the cheese melts.
4. This step works out well in the microwave, stirring every 2-3 min. to keep the sauce smooth.
5. Fold mixture, with macaroni, into a greased 2 qt. casserole dish.

Topping:

1 c. bread crumbs	2 Tbsp. melted margarine

6. Mix together and scatter over the top of the macaroni.
7. Bake uncovered for 30 min.

Serves 4-6 with salad and European wieners.

Cheesy Broccoli Rice Bake

So easy and so cheesy!

4 ½ c. cooked rice of choice (**wild rice** is nice!)
1 c. broccoli, chopped   4 Tbsp. butter
1 c. cauliflower, chopped   ½ onion, chopped
2 10 oz. cans creamed soup (celery or mushroom)
1 c. milk   1 10 oz. jar cheese whiz

1. Preheat oven to 350° F.
2. Cook rice; steam broccoli and cauliflower.
3. Sauté onion in butter.
4. Combine soup, milk and cheese.
5. Put all ingredients into a casserole dish.
6. Bake, uncovered, for 40- 50 min.

Serves 12 to 16. (the recipe can easily be halved)

Wild Rice Soup

Add some chicken for a complete meal or serve before a dinner of roast chicken on Sunday! (this soup can also be made for Monday to make use of the leftover roast chicken!)

¼ c. margarine	2 ½ c. wild rice, cooked
2 stalks of celery, sliced	2 c. water
2 carrots, grated	2 ¼ c. chicken broth
1 onion, chopped	2 c. fat-free evaporated milk
1 green pepper, chopped	2/3 c. slivered almonds, toasted
1/3 c. flour	½ tsp. pepper
½ c. fresh parsley, chopped	

1. Melt margarine in large saucepan, over med-high heat.
2. Cook celery, carrot, onion, and green pepper in the margarine —about 4 min., stirring occasionally, until tender.
3. Stir in flour and pepper, followed by wild rice, water and broth.
4. Heat to boiling; reduce heat to low, cover and simmer for 15 min., stirring occasionally.
5. Stir in evaporated milk, almonds, and parsley. Heat just until hot.

Serves 6 with Parmesan cheese/Garlic toast on top!

A great use of leftover wild rice! Sliced mushrooms can also be added.

Salads

Dressed Up Caesar Salad!

Mediterranean Pomegranate Salad

Oriental Coleslaw

Seven-Layer Summer Salad

Dressed Up Caesar Salad!

A great dinner salad for those hot summer nights when they appear!

½ c. caesar salad dressing
4 small chicken breasts, boneless skinless
1 head Romaine lettuce, torn up
½ c. croutons
¼ c. bacon bits
¼ c. Parmesan cheese, grated

1. Pour ¼ c. of the dressing over the chicken in a re-sealable plastic bag; turn to evenly coat the chicken. Refrigerate 30 min. to marinate.
2. Remove chicken from marinade, discard bag and marinade.
3. Preheat BBQ to med. heat. Grill chicken 5-7 min. on each side, or until cooked through (170 F.) Cut into thin slices.
4. Toss Romaine with remaining dressing, the chicken, croutons, bacon bits, and Parmesan.

Serves 4 with Foccacia, garlic toast or buns

Other additions: sliced cucumbers, mushrooms, cherry tomatoes

This recipe is also a great use of that Parmesan chicken you had on Sunday—save the leftovers to use in this salad for a weeknight. If there are leftovers from that combo—what a super lunch in a pita pocket or wrap!

Mediterranean Pomegranate Salad

Such a treat and good for you, too!

1 head Romaine lettuce, washed/torn

1 bunch Spinach leaves, stems removed, washed/torn

Seeds of 1 Pomegranate
(easy to remove: halve the pomegranate and place in a bowl of water while working the seeds out)

¼ c. pecans, chopped and toasted (toast in a pan on the stove top, stir and watch closely)

½ c. feta cheese, crumbled

Dressing:

1/3 c. olive oil	1 tsp. Dijon mustard
1 Tbsp. red wine vinegar	½ tsp. oregano
2 Tbsp. maple syrup	Sea salt and freshly ground pepper

1. Toss lettuce and spinach together in a large salad bowl.
2. Add pomegranate seeds, pecans, and feta cheese.
3. Whisk dressing ingredients together, store in fridge, and toss with salad just before serving.

Serves 6 and goes great with the Moroccan chicken!

Oriental Coleslaw

A great salad to add to that BBQ or mid-winter chicken wings—it really goes with everything!

1 pkg. ramen noodles (flavour of choice)　3 c. broccoli slaw
¼ c. slivered almonds　1 carrot, grated
3 c. cabbage slaw　½ apple, grated (unpeeled)
Dressing:
¼ c. canola oil　2 Tbsp. sugar
3 Tbsp. rice vinegar　1 seasoning pkg. from noodles

1. Pre-heat oven to 350° F.
2. Break up noodles, while still in pkg. ; spread out on baking sheet with almonds.
3. Toast in oven for 10 min., until lightly golden, stirring twice. Set aside to cool.
4. Toss the two slaws together in a medium bowl. Add the carrot, apple, and cooled noodle mixture; toss to combine.
5. For the **dressing**, shake the ingredients together in a jar and drizzle over the salad; toss to combine.
6. Serve immediately.

Serves 6

This salad goes well for leftovers the next day, but a third day is pushing it!

Seven-Layer Summer Salad

So colourful when made in a clear glass bowl!

4 c. spinach, torn	1 green pepper chopped
1 ½ c. mozzarella-cheddar mix, grated	½ c. light mayonnaise
2 c. mushrooms, sliced	½ c. light sour cream
1 small red onion, sliced	¼ c. chopped fresh basil
2 tomatoes, chopped	2 Tbsp. bacon bits

> *Other items can be added or substituted, such as cucumbers, broccoli, cauliflower, snow peas, pecans, feta cheese, dried cranberries*

1. Layer the spinach, 1 c. of the cheese, mushrooms, onion, tomatoes and green peppers in a 3 L. serving bowl.
2. Mix mayonnaise, sour cream, and basil. Spread over salad, completely covering the surface.
3. Cover and refrigerate at least 5 hours.
4. Sprinkle with remaining ½ c. cheese and the bacon bits just before serving.

Serves 12! (Serving size of 1 c. each —great for those big family BBQs!)

> *Want something smaller? Adjust quantities to serve 4, 6, or 8*
> *Serving sizes may end up being 2 c. each, so be sure to adjust for that as well!*

Breads

BBQ Bacon-Cheese Calzones

Cheddar Dumplings

Cheesy-Onion Sandwich Fold-overs

Easy Bruschetta

Grilled English Muffin Sandwiches

Sausage-Spinach Calzones

Stylish Bread Bowls

The Best Banana Bread

French Onion Biscuits

Zipped Up Cheese Bread

Herb's Focaccia

Italian French Bread

Mighty Naan Bread

Pepper Parmesan Breadsticks

Saturday Afternoon Cheddar Biscuits

So Simple Cheddar Beer Bread

Your Own Biscuit Mix

Your Own Biscuits

BBQ Bacon-Cheese Calzones

A different touch to a Saturday BBQ!

1 lb. pizza dough	½ small onion, chopped finely
1 Tbsp. extra-virgin olive oil	¾ lb. ground beef
¾ c. cheddar cheese, grated	4 slices bacon
Salt	2 tomatoes, chopped

1. Preheat BBQ to med-high.
2. Divide the pizza dough and form into 2 balls. Place in a large bowl, greased with 1 Tbsp. of the olive oil; cover with plastic wrap and let rest at room temp 15 min.
3. In a large skillet, cook the beef over med-high heat, breaking up the chunks, until browned—about 5 min. Drain and transfer to a large bowl.
4. In the same skillet, cook the bacon until crisp. Drain on paper towels. Reserve the drippings in the skillet.
5. Add the onion to the skillet and cook over medium heat, stirring occasionally, until softened—about 5 min; add to the beef in the bowl.
6. Crumble the bacon into the beef mixture and stir in the cheese; season with salt.
7. On a lightly floured surface, roll out 1 ball of the dough into a 12 inch round and transfer to a large oiled baking sheet.
8. Place half the beef mixture on one side of the round and top with half of the tomatoes.
9. Fold the dough in half over the filling, crimping the edge to seal.
10. Repeat with the remaining dough and filling.
11. Brush the calzones with olive oil; slice 2 vents into the top of each calzone.
12. Transfer the baking sheet to the BBQ, cover and bake until golden brown—about 20 min.

Serves 4 with salad (Caesar or Spinach)

Cheddar Dumplings

The perfect topper for that comforting stew!

1 ½ c. self-rising flour
½ tsp. ground mustard
2/3 c. milk

½ c. sharp cheddar cheese, grated
¼ c. shortening

1. In med. bowl, stir together flour and mustard
2. Cut in shortening, using pastry blender or fork, until mixture is crumbly.
3. Stir in cheese; add milk and stir just until mixture is moistened.
4. Drop dough by rounded spoonfuls onto simmering stew.
5. Cover and cook over med-low heat for 25 min., until dumplings are firm when pressed.

Serves 6—double recipe if you have a BIG stew.

These dumplings would be a great addition to a stew you saved, just to change it up for the second offering!

Cheesy-Onion Sandwich Fold-overs

A super sandwich for using leftovers!

4 tortillas	1/3 c. mayonnaise
2 Tbsp. extra-virgin olive oil	2 onions, sliced thin
2 c. shredded turkey (or chicken or ham)	
Salt and pepper	5 oz. baby spinach
8 oz. Pepper Jack cheese, grated	

1. Preheat the oven to 400F.
2. In a large skillet, heat 1 Tbsp. olive oil over medium heat.
3. Add the onions, sprinkle with salt and pepper, and cook, stirring occasionally, until soft and golden (about 10 min.)
4. Brush the tortillas with the remaining olive oil, and place on a baking sheet covered with parchment paper.
5. Bake the tortillas until browned—about 5 min.
6. In a medium bowl, stir together the cheese and mayonnaise; spread this mix on the tortillas and sprinkle the onions on top of the mix.
7. Bake until the cheese is bubbly—about 2 min.
8. Top the onions with the meat and bake for 5 min. more.
9. Add the spinach and fold the tortillas in half. Serve immediately.

Serves 4 with soup, salad, or veggies and dip.

Easy Bruschetta

A fun addition to a light meal or an appetizer for any meal

2 large garlic cloves, minced
¼ tsp. ea. of salt and pepper
1/3 c. extra virgin olive oil
½ Tbsp. dried basil
1 24" sourdough baguette
6-9 Roma tomatoes, chopped
¼ c. crumbled herb feta cheese (or mozzarella)

1. In a large bowl, combine garlic, salt, pepper, and a few drops of oil. Mash with a wooden spoon to make a paste.
2. Stir in the rest of the oil with tomatoes and basil and mix.
3. Preheat the broiler and cut bread into ½" to 3/4"slices.
4. Brush the top of each piece with olive oil and place under the broiler until golden brown.
5. Spoon tomato mixture onto each bread piece and broil until cheese starts to sizzle.

Try different additions such as prosciutto slices on the bread before the tomato mixture gets added.

Grilled English Muffin Sandwiches

Dressed up version to have with soup on a winter's night!

4 English muffins, split
8 slices preferred cheese
Salt and pepper

Margarine
1 large tomato, sliced

1. Heat a griddle over med-low heat.
2. Lightly spread each English muffin half with margarine.
3. Arrange the tomato and cheese slices on one half of each muffin.
4. Sprinkle with salt and pepper; assemble sandwiches together.
5. Place the sandwiches on the griddle and cook, turning once until cheese is melted and muffins are golden brown, about 8 min.

Serves 4 with soup of choice, or salad.

These sandwiches are also great with other fillings such as ham and cheese; tuna, salmon, or crab with cheese and tomato.

Sausage-Spinach Calzones

A great take-along lunch or fun supper

2 lb. baby spinach
½ lb. sweet Italian sausage, casings removed
2 Tbsp. extra-virgin olive oil
1 onion, chopped
1 ½ c. grated mozzarella cheese
1/4 c. grated parmesan cheese
Salt and pepper
1 lb. pizza dough
1 ½ c. marinara sauce

1. In a large skillet, bring ¼ c. water to a boil over med-high heat.
2. Add half of the spinach and cook, turning until wilted, 1 to 2 min., drain. Repeat with the remaining spinach. Let cool slightly, then squeeze to remove as much moisture as possible.
3. Coarsely chop the spinach, and then transfer to a large bowl.
4. In the same skillet, cook the sausage over med-high heat, breaking it up, until browned—about 5 min.
5. Add 1 Tbsp. olive oil with the onion and cook, scraping up any brown bits, until the onion is softened—about 5 min.
6. Transfer the sausage mixture to the spinach mixture. Stir in the mozzarella and parmesan, season with salt and pepper.
7. Preheat the oven to 425 F. Grease a baking sheet with 1 ½ tsp. olive oil. On the baking sheet, stretch out the dough to form a 10" x 15" rectangle. Place the filling mixture over the dough leaving a 1" border all around. Fold the 1" edges toward the centre, and then fold each long edge over the filling, covering the filling.
8. Flip the calzone seam side down and re-tuck any open ends.
9. Rub the remaining olive oil over the calzone, then cut 2 small vents in the top.
10. Bake until golden, 30 to 35 min. Cut into squares and serve with the marinara sauce.

Serves 6 with Caesar salad at dinner or heat up as is for lunch!

Stylish Bread Bowls

Chowders, chili, and stews are so special served in these bowls!

1 loaf (1 lb.) frozen bread dough, thawed	1 Tbsp. olive or canola oil
1 tsp. dried basil leaves	½ tsp. garlic powder

1. Spray outsides of six 10 oz. custard cups with canola spray.
2. Divide dough into 6 equal pieces. Shape each piece into a ball, then into a 6" round. Place rounds over bottom of custard cups.
3. Heat oven to 350° F.
4. Brush dough with oil; sprinkle on basil and garlic powder.
5. Cover and let rise in a warm place for 20 min.
6. Bake bowls for 20 min., or until golden brown.
7. Cool 5 min.; remove from cups and place right side up on wire rack. (inside of bowls may be slightly moist)
8. To serve, place warm or cooled bread bowls in shallow soup or pasta bowls; spoon in soup, chili or stew.

Serves 6 with the bread bowls all set to eat after the soup!

Sour cream and grated cheese are great to have ready on the side!

These bowls can be made during the last hour of the soup cooking, or make earlier in the day, or night before, and warm up before serving.

The Best Banana Bread

SO wonderful to come home to!

(and a great use of those poor ripe bananas!)

2 c. sugar	2 ½ c. flour
1 c. margarine	2 tsp. baking soda
6 ripe bananas	1 tsp. salt

> Bananas are easy to use if you keep them in the freezer; thaw when ready to use and the banana just slips right out of its skin!

1. Preheat oven to 350° F.
2. Cream margarine and sugar with electric beater, until light and fluffy.
3. Add bananas with eggs and beat until well mixed.
4. Sift dry ingredients 3 times.
5. Blend with banana mixture—do not over mix!
6. Pour into 2 loaf pans, sprayed with canola spray.
7. Bake for 45 min-1 hour; test for doneness.
8. Cool on rack for 10 min. before removing from the pans. Enjoy!

Makes 2 loaves, which freeze well—betcha you can only freeze one though—the first will be gone in a flash!

> 1/2 c. of chopped walnuts or pecans can be added. Kids LOVE chocolate chips to be added! This recipe can also be used for muffins—cut the baking time in half.

French Onion Biscuits

Super quick addition to your soup night!

2 c. biscuit mix
1 c. French onion dip
¼ c. milk

1. Preheat oven to 450 F.
2. In medium bowl, stir together all ingredients, until soft dough forms.
3. Drop dough into 6 mounds onto baking pan prepared with canola spray.
4. Bake 10 to 12 min. or until golden brown.
5. Serve warm.

Serves 6 with soup or stew. (great for dipping the biscuits!)

Other dips can be used in place of the French Onion Dip:

Herb and Garlic, Jalapeno and Cheddar
(very good—especially with the Taco Soup—Ola!)

Zipped-Up Cheese Bread

A great addition to soups and chowders!

2 c. flour	½ tsp. salt
1 c. buttermilk	¼ c. margarine, melted
1 c. grated Monterey Jack cheese with	Jalapeno peppers
1 tsp. sugar	2 eggs, slightly beaten
1 tsp. baking powder	½ tsp. baking soda

1. Preheat oven to 350° F.
2. Spray **bottom only** of loaf pan with canola spray; **spray well**
3. In a medium bowl, stir together flour, cheese, sugar, baking powder, baking soda, and salt.
4. Stir in remaining ingredients just until moistened—**batter should be lumpy**!
5. Spread batter in loaf pan.
6. Bake 35 to 45 min., or until golden brown and toothpick inserted in the center comes out clean.
7. Cool 5 min., run knife around edges of pan to loosen the bread, and turn out to a wire rack.
8. Cool 30 min. before slicing.

Serves 10-12 (maybe!)

Other cheeses can be used in place of the Monterey

Herb's Focaccia

Perfect addition to Chowder Night! (or salad night in the summer!)

¾ c. warm water
2 3/4 c. biscuit mix
4 tsp. olive oil
1 tsp. fresh oregano, chopped (or ½ tsp. dried)
1 pkg. quick active dry yeast
1/3 red onion, finely chopped

1. In a med. bowl, stir together water, yeast, biscuit mix, oregano, ¼ c. of the onion, and 3 tsp. of the oil (dough should be soft)
2. Place dough on surface sprinkled with biscuit mix, roll to coat.
3. Knead gently about 20 times, until smooth (add a bit of biscuit mix if dough sticks to surface)
4. Spray baking sheet with canola spray (or use parchment paper). Pat dough onto baking sheet into a 10" round. Sprinkle remaining onion onto dough's surface.
5. Brush remaining oil over onion and dough.
6. Cover and let rise in a warm place for 1 hour or until double (with 15 min. to go, heat oven to 400 F.)
7. Bake 12-15 min. or until light golden brown.
8. Immediately remove from baking sheet to wire rack. Serve warm or cooled. Cut into 12 wedges.

Serves 12 (or 6!) with chowder, stew, or chili.

Balsamic vinegar and olive oil is nice for dipping!

Italian French Bread

Perfect with your Swedish Meatballs!

1 loaf of French bread, cut lengthwise, through the middle, in half
½ c. creamy Caesar dressing   1 c. shredded mozzarella cheese

1. Preheat oven to 450 F.
2. Place bread halves on *ungreased* baking sheet.
3. Spread dressing on cut sides of the bread and sprinkle with cheese.
4. Bake 10-12 min., or until cheese is melted and edges are browning.
5. Cut into 12 serving pieces.
6. Serve warm.

Serves 12 with almost any entree, but especially good with soups and stews!

Mighty Naan Bread

Great as a side bread for casual dinners or as the base for pizza!

3 ½ to 4 c. flour	1 Tbsp. plain yogurt
1 tsp. baking powder	1 egg
1 tsp. sugar	1 ½ c. water
½ tsp. salt	

1. In a large bowl, mix dry ingredients together; make a well.
2. Add egg, yogurt, and water gradually; mix until dough comes firmly away from the sides of the bowl.
3. Knead dough on a floured board until the dough becomes elastic.
4. Pinch off pieces of dough about the size of a golf ball.
5. Place in a buttered pan, cover with a damp cloth and let sit for 1 hour. (may be refrigerated for several days at this point)
6. To bake: Preheat oven to 450 F. Form the balls into thin 4" diameter circles.
7. Place on a baking sheet and bake for 10 min., until puffy and golden brown.

Makes 25—30 pieces and can be served with Tzatziki sauce.

Small wedges go well as an appetizer! Herbs such as dried rosemary, basil, and parsley can be sprinkled on before baking.

Pepper-Parmesan Breadsticks

Super for the soup or spaghetti night!

2 c. Your Own Biscuit Mix (page 215)
½ c. cold water
1 Tbsp. margarine, melted
1/3 c. Parmesan cheese, shredded
½ tsp. fresh cracked pepper

1. Preheat oven to 450 F.
2. Prep a baking sheet with canola spray.
3. In a medium bowl, stir together biscuit mix, water, pepper and 2 Tbsp. of the cheese, until a soft dough forms.
4. Place dough on a surface sprinkled with biscuit mix; roll to coat.
    Roll into a 10" X 8" rectangle.
5. Brush rectangle with margarine and sprinkle with remaining cheese; press it in gently. Cut crosswise into 12 strips.
6. Gently twist the strips. Place ½ inch apart on the baking sheet.
7. Sprinkle strips with additional pepper.
8. Bake 10 to 12 min., until golden brown. Serve warm.

Serves 12 (or 6!) with soup, stew, chili, or spaghetti.

Saturday Afternoon Cheddar Biscuits

Add variety to your soup night—a snowy Saturday afternoon is perfect for making these biscuits!

(how can you tell I live in a place that has seen snow 10 months of the year ?!)

½ c. low-fat margarine
2 ½ c. grated old cheddar cheese
1 ¼ c. flour
½ tsp. salt

2 tsp. lemon pepper
1 Tbsp. parsley
2 Tbsp. sesame seeds

1. Cream margarine until soft and fluffy.
2. Add cheese and mix well.
3. Combine flour, salt, lemon pepper and parsley; add to cheese mixture.
4. Mix until dough just holds together.
5. Divide dough into two parts; roll into 2 logs, 1" in diameter.
6. Roll logs in sesame seeds to coat.
7. Freeze for 30 min. to make cutting easier.
8. Preheat oven to 375° F.
9. Cut logs into ¼" thick slices and place slices on *ungreased* baking sheets, 2" apart.
10. Bake for 12 to 15 min., or until just golden. Cool on wire rack.

Makes about 48 biscuits—do not count on them all making it to dinner time!

So Simple Cheddar Beer Bread

Now say that 5 times real fast! By the time you get that right, the bread will be done, ready to serve with some wonderful soup!

3 c. flour	2 c. grated sharp cheddar cheese
1 Tbsp. baking powder	½ onion, finely chopped
¾ tsp. salt	3 garlic cloves, minced
2 Tbsp. sugar	12 oz. can of beer

1. Preheat oven to 350° F.
2. Combine all the ingredients, up to the beer, in a bowl and stir with a fork, until well mixed.
3. Add the beer, ¼ at a time, until all the ingredients are blended.
4. Spoon into a 4" x 8" loaf pan that has been sprayed with canola spray; smooth down with a spatula.
5. Bake for one hour; remove from pan and cool on a wire rack.

Serves 8 to 10—perfect with **Hamburger Soup!**

Did your neighbour give you some zucchini this past summer? Put in 1 c. cheese and 1 c. grated zucchini!

Your Own Biscuit Mix

So handy when a biscuit mix is called for in a recipe and it is also ready in a jiffy when quick biscuits are needed at supper time!

8 c. flour
6 Tbsp. baking powder
2 Tbsp. cream of tartar
¼ c. sugar

1 lb shortening
1 ¼ c. powdered milk
1 ½ Tbsp. salt

1. In large bowl, combine all dry ingredients.
2. Cut in shortening, using pastry blender or fork, until mixture is crumbly.
3. Place mixture in container with airtight lid and store in the pantry until needed.

> This mixture can be stored for months at room temperature and is ready to use for biscuits and pancakes.

Your Own Biscuits

Quick biscuits with Your Own Biscuit Mix!

3 c. Your Own Biscuit Mix 1 c. grated cheese (optional)
¾ c. water

1. Pre-heat oven to 450 F.
2. Blend all ingredients and knead on floured board 10 times.
3. Drop by teaspoonfuls onto cookie sheet.
4. Bake at 450 F. for 10 min.

Makes 1 dozen (may need to double the recipe to have some for the freezer!)

Breakfast

Sleepover French Toast

Overnight Cinnamon Buns

Your Own Pancakes

Breakfast Smoothies

Your Smoothie Recipe

No-Bake Chewy Nutty Granola Fruit Bars

Sleepover French Toast

Prepped the night before makes your AM so organized!

12 eggs
½ c. cream
2 Tbsp. Orange liqueur or orange juice
Loaf French bread, sliced 1" thick
Zest of 1 orange
½ tsp. vanilla

1. In bowl, whisk together eggs, cream, vanilla, orange zest, and liqueur.
2. Place sliced bread in 9" x 13" pan; pour egg mixture over bread; be sure that bread is well coated.
3. Cover with lid or plastic wrap and place in fridge overnight.
4. In the AM, preheat oven to 375° F.
5. Place bread slices on baking sheet sprayed with canola spray
6. Bake for 20 to 25 min.

Serves 6 with fruit and maple syrup with sausages on the side!

Overnight Cinnamon Buns

A great breakfast item for sleepovers and family get-togethers —prep the night before and pop into the oven the next AM, one half hour before those sleepy eyes appear in the kitchen!

15 frozen dough rolls	2 Tbsp. cinnamon
¾ c. brown sugar	¼ c. melted butter
¼ c. instant vanilla pudding powder	
¾ c. chopped pecans (and/or raisins)	

1. Prep a bundt pan with canola spray.
2. Add frozen dough rolls; place sideways and layered.
3. Sprinkle with brown sugar, pudding powder, cinnamon and pecans.
4. Pour melted butter overall; cover with a clean, damp cloth.
5. The next AM, preheat oven to 350° F. and bake for 25 min. (place a baking sheet on **bottom of oven** to catch any drips)
6. Let sit for 5 min.; turn out onto a serving plate.

Serves 8 to 10 with a fruit tray.

Our family especially loves this on a ski weekend!
It is easy to make just about anywhere!

Your Own Pancakes

Zip these up quick Sunday AM with Your Own Biscuit Mix!

3 c. Your Own Biscuit Mix   1 ¼ c. water
1 egg

1. Grease griddle with 1 tsp. canola oil and pre-heat to 350° F.
2. Blend all ingredients with wire whisk—just until mixed—**should still be lumpy!**
3. Griddle is ready when a drop of water sizzles.
4. Use ladle to drop batter on griddle—turn pancakes with metal spatula when bubbles appear on the surface.
5. Pancakes are ready when steam stops from the bottom surface.
6. As you make the pancakes, keep them warm in the oven until all are done.

Makes 18 medium sized pancakes served with pancake syrup and preferred toppings; a side of sausages and fruit completes the breakfast! (could be supper also!)

Breakfast Smoothies

Zap a nutritious breakfast together—prep your blender the night before, with ingredients all set to go at the front of your fridge—you can do this in your sleep!

1 banana, in pieces	6-8 strawberries, halved
½ grapefruit, in pieces	½ c. milk
1 Tbsp. wheat germ	2 tsp. flax seed
½ tsp. vanilla	

1. Place all ingredients in the blender and process until smooth.

Makes 2 servings.

Try blueberries in place of the strawberries—makes a great purple drink!
Experiment with various fruits to find your favourite blend!
Yogurt can also be added.

Your Smoothie Recipe

Just adjust the ingredients with the proportions balanced and you have your own customized smoothie —all set for the day!

1 ½ c. skim milk	1 c. frozen strawberries
½ c. peaches	2 Tbsp. frozen orange juice
½ c. vanilla low-fat yogurt	½ c. ice cubes

1. Blend all ingredients until smooth; enjoy!

Serves 2-3

Other choices of fruit:

Blueberries, mangoes, watermelon, banana (nice thickener that goes well with just about anything else), apple juice, raspberries, blackberries, pineapple, nectarines, plums

Other healthy additions to try:

1 Tbsp. wheat germ, 2 tsp. flax seeds, 2 tsp. bran

2-3 handfuls of green leafy vegetable such as spinach (really!)

No-Bake Chewy Nutty Granola Fruit Bars

These are great when having yogurt for breakfast, mid-morning snack, supplement to lunch, mid-afternoon snack, evening snack: just about any time!

1 ¼ c. old-fashioned oats	¼ tsp. ground cinnamon
1 c. (5 oz.) cashews	3 Tbsp. light corn syrup
3 Tbsp. (1 ½ oz.) unsalted butter	1 Tbsp. molasses
½ c. dark brown sugar	½ tsp. coarse salt

> **Options:** Cashews can be any combination of 1 c. nuts ie. Almonds, pecans, sunflower seeds, flax seeds, pumpkin seeds; craisins, raisins or any other dried fruit can be combined with the oats to make 1 ¼ c.

1. Line a 4 ½ by 9 inch loaf pan with plastic wrap, leaving a 1 inch overhang on each long side.
2. Toast oats and nuts in a large skillet, stirring often until aromatic and just starting to turn golden brown. (5—6 min.) Transfer to a medium bowl.
3. Add butter, sugar, cinnamon, corn syrup, molasses, and salt in the skillet; cook over medium heat, stirring until butter melts and mixture bubbles. (2-3 min.) Pour hot mixture over the oats mixture, in the bowl, and stir to combine.
4. Transfer mixture to the loaf pan. Using a spatula, press mixture into an even layer. Refrigerate until set (about 30 min.—it is okay to wait until the next day, as well)
5. Remove chilled mixture from the pan using the plastic to lift it out. Discard the plastic and cut into ¾ or 1 inch thick bars.
6. Store in an airtight container with parchment paper between the bars so they do not stick together.

Treats

Gingerbread Bundt Cake

Heavenly Strawberry Dessert

Nuts for Sweet and Spicy

Gingerbread Bundt Cake

A warm and cozy winter dessert!

2 tsp. ginger	½ tsp. cloves
1 tsp. baking powder	2 eggs
¾ tsp. baking soda	1 c. molasses
½ tsp. salt	2/3 c. canola oil
½ tsp. cinnamon	1 c. water
½ tsp. nutmeg	2 c. flour
1 c. sugar	¼ c. unsweetened cocoa

1. Pre-heat oven to 350° F.
2. Spray Bundt pan with canola spray; sprinkle with flour.
3. In large bowl, mix flour, sugar, cocoa, ginger, baking powder, baking soda, salt, cinnamon, nutmeg, and cloves; mix well.
4. In medium bowl, lightly beat eggs; add molasses and oil; beat well.
5. Stir water into egg mixture.
6. Add egg mixture to flour mixture; beat just until combined.
7. Pour batter into sprayed and floured pan.
8. Bake for 45-60 min., or until toothpick comes out clean.
9. Cool in pan on wire rack for 15 min.; invert onto serving plate.
10. Cool 30 min., or until completely cooled.
11. Just before serving, dust with powdered sugar.

Heavenly Strawberry Dessert

A wonderful finish to a summer BBQ!

2 c. graham cracker crumbs	½ c. strawberry jam
1/3 c. low-fat margarine	16 fresh strawberries, chopped
3 c. whipped topping, thawed	1 c. plus 2 Tbsp. sugar

4 pkg.(250 g. ea.) light brick cream cheese, softened

1. Mix graham crumbs and margarine; press onto bottom of 13" x 9" pan. Refrigerate while preparing filling.
2. In a large bowl, beat cream cheese and 1 c. sugar with electric mixer until well blended. Add jam; mix well.
3. In a small bowl, place strawberries and remaining 2 Tbsp. sugar; stir well to mix.
4. Stir strawberries and whipped topping into cream cheese mixture. Spoon over crust and cover.
5. Refrigerate for 4 hours, or until firm.

Serves 20 (!) with one piece each. Saves well for next day's meal.

Option: cut recipe in half to make only half the amount

Nuts for Sweet and Spicy

Perfect for Holiday times!

2 egg whites	1/2 tsp. cinnamon
2 tsp. brown sugar	2 c. mixed nut mixture
1 tsp. pumpkin pie spice	(cashews, almonds, etc.)

1. Pre-heat oven to 350° F.
2. In medium bowl, beat egg whites and spices together until frothy.
3. Stir in nuts—cover well.
4. Spread nuts onto parchment paper-covered baking sheet.
5. Bake 15 min., or until nuts are almost dry-looking (stir halfway through) Cool completely.

Makes 2 cups—multiply ingredients as needed. For gifts, place into decorative jars or tins.

Add other ingredients such as currents or craisins for additional festive flavour!

Recipe Index

Recipe Index

Beef

A S*low* Beef Roll in Italy, 97
Beef Burgers—All Cheesed-Up!, 121
Beef Fajitas BBQ Flavour, 122
Beefy Burritos, 124
Beefy Meatballs, 98
Cheddar Beef Tortiere, 125
Cheesy Beef Burgers, 126
Coffee-Seasoned Steaks, 127
Easier than Lasagna Burgers, 128
Great Caesar Burgers, 130
Italian Beef and Ravioli Stew, 132
Mushroom Beef Dip, 113
Rouladen S*low* Dance, 99
Savoury Pot Roast with Mushroom Sauce, 103
Southwestern Fajitas, 138
Tanged up Beef Patties, 123
Truly Divine Meatloaf, 131
Zesty Taco Pie, 133

Bread

Herb's Focaccia, 209

Breads

BBQ Bacon-Cheese Calzones, 199
Cheddar Dumplings, 200
Cheesy-Onion Sandwich Fold-overs, 201
Easy Bruschetta, 202
French Onion Biscuits, 207
Grilled English Muffin Sandwiches, 203
Italian French Bread, 210
Mighty Naan Bread, 211
Pepper-Parmesan Breadsticks, 212
Saturday Afternoon Cheddar Biscuits, 213
Sausage-Spinach Calzones, 204
So Simple Cheddar Beer Bread, 214
Stylish Bread Bowls, 205
The Best Banana Bread, 206
Your Own Biscuit Mix, 215
Your Own Biscuits, 216
Zipped-Up Cheese Bread, 208

Breakfast

Breakfast Smoothies, 224
No-Bake Chewy Nutty Granola Fruit Bars, 226
Overnight Cinnamon Buns, 222
Sleepover French Toast, 221
Your Own Pancakes, 223
Your Smoothie Recipe, 225

Chicken/Turkey

Almond-Dijon Baked Chicken, 139
BBQ Honey-Mustard Chicken Thighs, 140
Chicken Chowder, 101
Chicken Cordon Bleu, Made Easy, 141
Cozy-all-over Moroccan Chicken, 142
El Spicy Chicken and Rice, 108
Fiesta-to-the-Max Chicken Enchiladas, 143
Fresh Veggie-Chicken BBQ Kebabs, 144
Herbed Chicken, 111
Roast Herbed Chicken and Vegetables, 137
Southwestern Fajitas, 138
Spicy Citrus Chicken, 104
Teriyaki Chicken with Orange Sauce, 105
Turkey Sausage and Tortellini Soup, 106
Turkey, Mushroom and Rice Soup, 107

Fish/Seafood

Almond-Encrusted Tilapia, 175
Clammed-up Chowder, 176
Fishy Tomato Soup, 177
Grilled Salmon, 178
Ola! Crab Enchiladas, 179
SO Cool Crab Cakes, 181
Wild Rice Stuffed Salmon, 182

Pork

All Cheesy Ham and Eggs, 168
Cranberry–Orange Pork Chops on the S*low* Side, 159
Fiesta Peppered Sausage Burritos, 171
Ham and Cheese Frittata, 169
Orange-Dijonned Pork Chops, 114
Pork and Mushroom Marengo, 115
Pork Chops on Bed of Corn Bread Stuffing and Broccoli Mix, 166
So Good Spiced Ham Slices, 170
Stuffed and Wrapped Pork Chops, 167

Rice & Pasta

Cheesy Broccoli Rice Bake, 186
THE BEST Macaroni and Cheese!, 185
Wild Rice Soup, 187

Salads

Dressed Up Caesar Salad!, 191
Mediterranean Pomegranate Salad, 192
Oriental Coleslaw, 193
Seven-Layer Summer Salad, 194

S*low*-Cooker Recipes

A S*low* Beef Roll in Italy, 97
Basil Italian Sausage Lasagna, 100
Beefy Meatballs, 98
Chicken Chowder, 101
Cranberry–Orange Pork Chops on the S*low* Side, 159
Crazy-Nutty Mocha Pudding Cake, 102
El Spicy Chicken and Rice, 108
French Onion Soup, 109
Hearty Sausage Casserole, 110
Herbed Chicken, 111
Hunter Sausage Casserole, 112
Mushroom Beef Dip, 113
Orange-Dijonned Pork Chops, 114
Pork and Mushroom Marengo, 115
Rouladen S*low* Dance, 99
Savoury Pot Roast with Mushroom Sauce, 103
Spicy Citrus Chicken, 104
Taco Soup, 116
Teriyaki Chicken with Orange Sauce, 105
Turkey Sausage and Tortellini Soup, 106
Turkey, Mushroom and Rice Soup, 107

Soups

French Onion Soup, 109
Taco Soup, 116
Turkey Sausage and Tortellini Soup, 106
Turkey, Mushroom and Rice Soup, 107

Treats

Crazy-Nutty Mocha Pudding Cake, 102
Gingerbread Bundt Cake, 231
Heavenly Strawberry Dessert, 232
Nuts for Sweet and Spicy, 233

Printed in Great Britain
by Amazon